Lecture Notes in Computational Vision and Biomechanics

Volume 13

For further volumes:
http://www.springer.com/series/8910

The research related to the analysis of living structures (Biomechanics) has been a source of recent research in several distinct areas of science, for example, Mathematics, Mechanical Engineering, Physics, Informatics, Medicine and Sport. However, for its successful achievement, numerous research topics should be considered, such as image processing and analysis, geometric and numerical modelling, biomechanics, experimental analysis, mechanobiology and enhanced visualization, and their application to real cases must be developed and more investigation is needed. Additionally, enhanced hardware solutions and less invasive devices are demanded.

On the other hand, Image Analysis (Computational Vision) is used for the extraction of high level information from static images or dynamic image sequences. Examples of applications involving image analysis can be the study of motion of structures from image sequences, shape reconstruction from images and medical diagnosis. As a multidisciplinary area, Computational Vision considers techniques and methods from other disciplines, such as Artificial Intelligence, Signal Processing, Mathematics, Physics and Informatics. Despite the many research projects in this area, more robust and efficient methods of Computational Imaging are still demanded in many application domains in Medicine, and their validation in real scenarios is matter of urgency.

These two important and predominant branches of Science are increasingly considered to be strongly connected and related. Hence, the main goal of the LNCV&B book series consists of the provision of a comprehensive forum for discussion on the current state-of-the-art in these fields by emphasizing their connection. The book series covers (but is not limited to):

- Applications of Computational Vision and Biomechanics
- Biometrics and Biomedical Pattern Analysis
- Cellular Imaging and Cellular Mechanics
- Clinical Biomechanics
- Computational Bioimaging and Visualization
- Computational Biology in Biomedical Imaging
- Development of Biomechanical Devices
- Device and Technique Development for Biomedical Imaging
- Experimental Biomechanics
- Gait & Posture Mechanics
- Grid and High Performance Computing for Computational Vision and Biomechanics
- Image Processing and Analysis
- Image Processing and Visualization in Biofluids
- Image Understanding
- Material Models

- Mechanobiology
- Medical Image Analysis
- Molecular Mechanics
- Multi-Modal Image Systems
- Multiscale Biosensors in Biomedical Imaging
- Multiscale Devices and Biomems for Biomedical Imaging
- Musculoskeletal Biomechanics
- Multiscale Analysis in Biomechanics
- Neuromuscular Biomechanics
- Numerical Methods for Living Tissues
- Numerical Simulation
- Software Development on Computational Vision and Biomechanics
- Sport Biomechanics
- Virtual Reality in Biomechanics
- Vision Systems

João Manuel R. S. Tavares
Xiongbiao Luo · Shuo Li
Editors

Bio-Imaging and Visualization for Patient-Customized Simulations

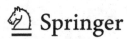 Springer

Editors
João Manuel R. S. Tavares
Faculdade de Engenharia
Universidade do Porto
Porto
Portugal

Shuo Li
GE Healthcare and University of Western
  Ontario
London, ON
Canada

Xiongbiao Luo
Graduate School of Information Science
Nagoya University
Nagoya
Japan

ISSN 2212-9391
ISBN 978-3-319-38087-2
DOI 10.1007/978-3-319-03590-1
Springer Cham Heidelberg New York Dordrecht London

ISSN 2212-9413 (electronic)
ISBN 978-3-319-03590-1 (eBook)

Preface

Imaging and Visualization are among the most dynamic and innovative areas of research of the past few decades. Justification of this activity arises from the requirements of important practical applications such as the visualization of computational data, the processing of medical images for assisting medical diagnosis and intervention, and the 3D geometry reconstruction and processing for computer simulations.

Currently, due to the development of more powerful hardware resources, mathematical and physical methods, investigators have been incorporating advanced computational techniques to derive sophisticated methodologies that can better enable the solution of the problems encountered. Consequent to these efforts any effective methodologies have been proposed, validated, and some of them have already been integrated into commercial software for computer simulations.

The main goal of the workshop *Bio-Imaging and Visualization for Patient-Customized Simulations*, that was organized under the auspicious of the *16th International Conference on Medical Image Computing and Computer Assisted Intervention (MICCAI 2013)*, held from September 22nd to 26th, 2013 in Nagoya, Japan, was to provide a platform for communications among specialists from complementary fields such as signal and image processing, mechanics, computational vision, mathematics, physics, informatics, computer graphics, bio-medical practice, psychology, and industry. Participants in this workshop presented and discussed their proposed techniques and methods and explored the translational potentials of these emerging technological fields. As such, an excellent forum was established to refine ideas for future work and to define constructive cooperation for new and improved solutions of imaging and visualization techniques and modeling methods toward more realistic and efficient computer simulations, between software developers, specialist researchers, and applied end-users from diverse fields related to signal processing, imaging, visualization, biomechanics, and simulation.

This book contains the full papers presented at the *MICCAI 2013* workshop *Bio-Imaging and Visualization for Patient-Customized Simulations (MWBIVPCS 2013)*. MWBIVPCS 2013 brought together researchers representing several fields, such as Biomechanics, Engineering, Medicine, Mathematics, Physics, and Statistic. The works included in this book present and discuss new trends in those fields, using several methods and techniques, including the finite element method, similarity metrics, optimization processes, graphs, Hidden Markov models, sensor calibration, fuzzy logic, data mining, cellular automation, active shape models, template matching, and level sets, in order to address more efficiently different and timely applications involving signal and image acquisition, image processing and analysis, image segmentation, image registration and fusion, computer simulation, image-based modeling, simulation and surgical planning, image-guided robot-assisted surgical, and image-based diagnosis.

The editors wish to thank all the *MWBIVPCS 2013* authors and members of the Program Committee for sharing their expertise, and also to *The MICCAI Society* for having hosted and supported the workshop within *MICCAI 2013*.

João Manuel R. S. Tavares
Xiongbiao Luo
Shuo Li

Workshop Organizers

João Manuel R. S. Tavares   Faculdade de Engenharia, Universidade do Porto
Porto, Portugal
Email: tavares@fe.up.pt
URL: www.fe.up.pt/~tavares

Xiongbiao Luo   Nagoya University
Nagoya, Japan
Email: xbluo@mori.m.is.nagoya-u.ac.jp
URL: http://www.mori.m.is.nagoya-u.ac.jp/~xbluo/

Shuo Li   University of Western Ontario
London, Canada Email: shuo.li@ge.com
URL: http://dig.lhsc.on.ca/members/shuo.php

Workshop Program Committee

Alberto Santamaria-Pang	GE Global Research Center, USA
Alexandre X. Falcão	Universidade Estadual de Campinas, Brazil
Aly Farag	Louisville University, USA
Bernard Gosselin	University of Mons, Belgium
Begoña Calvo	University of Zaragoza, Spain
Bin Gu	University of Western Ontario, Canada
Christos E. Constantinou	Stanford University, USA
Daniela Iacoviello	Università degli Studi di Roma "La Sapienza", Italy
Eduardo Soudah	International Center for Numerical Methods in Engineering, Spain
F. Xavier Roca	Universitat Autònoma de Barcelona, Spain
Francisco P. M. Oliveira	Universidade do Porto, Portugal
João Paulo Papa	Universidade Estadual Paulista, Brazil
Jorge Barbosa	Universidade do Porto, Portugal
Jorge S. Marques	Instituto Superior Técnico, Portugal
Josef Šlapal	Brno University of Technology, Czech Republic
Jack Yao	National Institutes of Health, USA
Joachim Hornegger	Friedrich-Alexander University Erlangen-Nuremberg, Germany
Jun Zhao	Shanghai Jiao Tong University, China
Khan M. Iftekharuddin	Old Dominion University, USA
Cristian A. Linte	Mayo Clinic, USA
M. Emre Celebi	Louisiana State University in Shreveport, USA
Manuel González Hidalgo	Balearic Islands University, Spain
Marc Thiriet	Universite Pierre et Marie Curie (Paris VI), France
Paolo Di Giamberardino	Sapienza University of Rome, Italy
Renato Natal Jorge	Universidade do Porto, Portugal
Reneta Barneva	State University of New York Fredonia, USA
Sanderson L. Gonzaga de Oliveira	Universidade Federal de Lavras, Brazil
Sandra Rua Ventura	Instituto Politécnico do Porto, Portugal
Victor Hugo C. de Albuquerque	Universidade de Fortaleza, Brazil

Acknowledgments

The editors wish to acknowledge:

- The MICCAI Society
- Universidade do Porto
- Faculdade de Engenharia, Universidade do Porto
- Fundação para a Ciência e a Tecnologia
- Instituto de Engenharia Mecânica e Gestão Industrial
- Nagoya University
- GE Healthcare Worldwide
- Digital Imaging Group of London
- University of Western Ontario
- Taylor & Francis Group
- Springer

for the support given in the organization of this MICCAI 2013 workshop on Bio-Imaging and Visualization for Patient-Customized Simulations.

Contents

A Novel Colon Wall Flattening Model
for Computed Tomographic Colonography:
Method and Validation

**Huafeng Wang, Lihong Li, Hao Han, Yunhong Wang, Weifeng Lv,
Xianfeng Gu and Zhengrong Liang**

Abstract Computed tomographic colonography (CTC) has been developed for
diagnosis of colon cancer. Flattening the three-dimensional (3D) colon wall into two-
dimensional (2D) image is believed to be much effective for providing supplementary
information to the endoscopic views and further facilitating colon registration, taniae
coli (TC) detection, and haustral folds segmentation. Though the previously-used
conformal mapping-based flattening methods can preserve the angle, it has limitations in providing accurate information of the 3D inner colon wall due to the lack of
undulating topography. In this paper, we present a novel colon wall flattening method
based on a 2.5D approach. Coupling with the conformal flattening model, the new
approach builds an elevation distance map to depict the neighborhood characteristics of the inner colon wall. We validated the new method via two CTC applications:

H. Wang (✉) · H. Han · Z. Liang
Department of Radiology, Stony Brook University, Stony Brook, NY, USA
e-mail: Wanghuafengbuaa@gmail.com

H. Wang
School of Software, Beihang University of Beijing, Beijing, China

L. Li
College of Staten Island, Victory Blvd, NY, USA
e-mail: lihong.li@csi.cuny.edu

Y. Wang · W. Lv
School of Computer Science, Beihang University Of Beijing, Beijing, China
e-mail: yhwang@buaa.edu.cn

X. Gu
Dept. of Computer Science, Stony Brook University, Stony Brook , NY, USA
e-mail: gu@cs.sunysb.edu

Z. Liang
e-mail: lihong.li@csi.cuny.edu

H. Han
e-mail: haohan@mil.sunysb.edu

J. M. R. S. Tavares et al. (eds.), *Bio-Imaging and Visualization for Patient-Customized
Simulations*, Lecture Notes in Computational Vision and Biomechanics 13,
DOI: 10.1007/978-3-319-03590-1_1, © Springer International Publishing Switzerland 2014

TC detection and haustral fold segmentation. Experimental results demonstrated the effectiveness of our model for CTC studies.

Keywords Conformal mapping · 2.5D representation · Colon wall · Medical imaging · Computed tomographic colonography

1 Introduction

According to the recent statistics from American Cancer Society (ACS) [1], colorectal cancer ranks the third most common occurrence of both cancer deaths and new cancer cases for both men and women in the United States. Early detection and removal of colonic polyps prior to their malignant transformation can effectively decrease the incidence of colon cancer [2]. As a new minimally-invasive screening technique, computed tomographic colonography (CTC) has shown several advantages over the traditional optical colonoscopy (OC).

In order to better depict the internal structure of the colon, traditional paradigm em-ploys CTC to achieve the tasks of screening and diagnosis. It utilizes endoscopic views to visualize the colon wall [3, 4]. It has been successfully demonstrated to be more convenient and efficient than the optical colonoscopy. However, due to the length and winding of colon structures, inspecting the entire colon wall is still time consuming and prone to cause errors by current CTC technologies. Moreover, the field-of-view (FOV) of the endoscopic views has limitations, and incomplete examinations are often observed.

Flattening the three-dimensional (3D) wall into two-dimensional (2D) image is be-lieved to be much effective for increasing the field of view (FOV) and providing supplementary information to the endoscopic views [5]. It is also an efficient visualization tool for polyp detection, in which the entire inner surface of the colon is dissected and flattened on a 2D plane. The flattened colon can be efficiently volume rendered to produce an electronic biopsy image for computer aided detection (CAD) of polyps [6]. Therefore, various flattening techniques [2, 5, 7, 8] have been studied, in which the conformal mapping algorithm [8] showed advantages in generating 2D colon wall with minimal distortion by preserving all the angles. An overview of colon flattening or unfolding approaches has listed in Table 1. Conformal mapping algorithm aims at preserving the local shape on the flattened colon surface. Hence it is high recommended for that the colon polyps usually have a semi-ellipsoidal shape which we want to preserve.

However, 2D flattening is capable of grasp the whole plate view at the cost of losing or distorting fine details, e.g., the relative height information among neighborhood of colon structure. For polyp diagnosis, the height variations of colon structure are usually of much value for judging the abnormity of tissue. Hence, we developed a novel 2.5D colon wall flattening method which will best describe not only the whole map of colon structure but also fine details of neighborhood of the components on the colon wall.

Table 1 Overview of the colon flattening or unfolding approaches

Authors	Technique	Strengths	Limitations	Year
Paik et al. [9]	Sampling the solid angle of the camera, and mapping it onto a cylinder	Straightforward	2D. It may cause distortions in shape	2000
Haker et al. [10]	Employing certain angle-preserving mappings	Presented a surface scan of the entire colon	2D. It requires a highly accurate and smooth surface mesh for a good mean-curvature calculation	2000
Bartrolf et al. [11]	Moving a camera along the central path of the colon (angle preserved)	Frame by frame, and intuitive	2D. It does not provide a complete overview of the colon	2001
Bartroli et al. [12]	Nonlinear unfolding and area preserving methods	Reduced the distortion that can result from this projection	Computational consume is large	2001
Wang et al. [13]	Exploring a volume-based flattening strategy	Volume-based. It considered the partial volume (PV) effect and preserves the original image intensity distribution	The distance-based mapping may not be accurate enough for detection of small polyps	2005
Hong et al. [5]	Utilizing conformal structure to flatten the colon wall onto a planar image. (angle preserved)	Minimized the global distortion	The de-noise algorithm cannot always get genus 0 surface	2006
Authors	Volumetric Curved Planar	Used volume rendering for hollow regions and standard CPR for the surrounding tissue	Curved Planar Reformation CPR and volume rendering are tightly coupled	2008
Jin et al. [14]	Discrete Ricci Flow	Minimized the global distortion, which means the local shape is well preserved	The gradient descending algorithm is not invariant by calculating the first order derivative	2008
Wei et al. [15]	Using Quasi-Conformal Mapping	Exploited the texture information	The quasi-conformal mapping deforms the circles to ellipses	2010
Yao et al. [16]	Using local projections	Preserved not only the topology of the original surface, but also the vertex resolution	The polyp and haustral folds size will be deformed by a constant angle sampling	2010

The remainder of this paper is organized as follows. The new colon flatten methodology is presented in Sect. 2. To validate the model, two application scenarios are presented in Sect. 3. In Sect. 4, discussions and conclusion about the new model are given. However, 2D is capable of grasp the whole plate view at the cost of losing or distorting some details. For example the relative height among neighborhood. Regarding the diagnosis, the height variances are usually of much value for judging the abnormity of tissue. On the contrary, our proposed technology will best describe not only the whole map of colon but also the details of neighborhood of the components on the colon wall.

2 Method

2.1 Overview of the Pipeline of 2.5D Colon Flattening Model

For the acquired CTC datasets, the first task is to segment the data volume and extract the colon wall as a volumetric mucosa (VM). This is achieved by a statistical maximum a posteriori expectation-maximization (MAP-EM) algorithm [17]. Considering the use of positive-contrast tagging agents to opacify the residual fecal for differentiation of the materials from colon wall, partial volume effects (PVE) became severe and the thickness of the VM varied dramatically. Because there exists PVE in CT scans which make the surface of colon wall more implicit, a levelset based shrinkage method will help to evolve a much better approximated mucosa surface inner the colon wall. In order to extract a polygonal mesh of an iso-surface from the 3D voxels, a marching cube process is introduced into the pipeline. Consequently, a more vividly described colon wall will be presented. In order to build a bridge connecting the 3D wall with the 2.5D morphological map, an inner wall cylinder model will be exploited and a distance map will be created according to the shortest distance map measured between the voxelized points and the given cylindrical surface. Hence, the 2.5D map of colon wall will exhibit geometric features which particularly conserve the original angle and the morphological shape to full extent. Figure 1 illustrates the whole pipeline of the 2.5D flattening model.

2.2 Level-Set Based Shrinkage to Initialize the Layer of Colon Wall(Shrinkage)

The starting layer (SL) is of much importance to describe the contour of the colon wall. We introduce the level set method [18] to retrieve a better SL, from which we build the distance transform to distinguish different topological structures. Compared with other methods, it is able to combine region-based information and edge-based information together, make use of global information and local information simultaneously and control the geometric property of level set function easily.

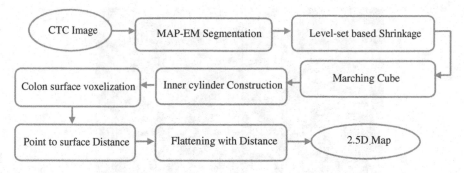

Fig. 1 The pipeline of the new method

Straightforwardly, it should reside inside the outermost and innermost layers, where the variation of CT intensities across the different layers remains relatively stable. Furthermore, the gradient of image intensity is used to construct the stopping criteria to stop the curve evolution by

$$\phi_t = \delta(\phi) \cdot \frac{\lambda}{1 + \|\nabla I\|} \{\alpha_0 A + \alpha_1 B + \alpha_2 C + \alpha_3 \text{div}(\nabla\phi/\|\nabla\phi\|)\} \qquad (1)$$

where ϕ is the Lipschitz function, and I represents the image intensity. The two superscripts in and out indicate the regions where $\Phi > 0$ and $\Phi \leq 0$ respectively, while A, B and C represent the square of the variance of the mean intensity values of voxels in the whole image, the narrow band and the local neighborhood respectively. The notations $\lambda, \alpha_0, \alpha_1, \alpha_2$ and α_3 are constants used to control the influence of each term, and ∇ represents the gradient operator. The div $(*)$ is the curvature of Lipschitz function, which control the smoothness of the zero level set surface.

Once the above evolution procedure stops (Eq. (1) converges), the resulting zero level set surface, where $\Phi_t = 0$, indicates a layer between the outermost and innermost layers where the variation of CT intensities changes slightly across different layers. As a result, we will get a series of voxels which represent the SL of the colon wall. Figure 2 illustrates the colon mesh after the marching cube process.

2.3 Building Distance Map with a Cylinder Model

To build a reliable cylinder model, relying on which we calculate the distance map (as shown in Fig. 3), we need to perform two things: (1) determination of the centerline (also known as medial or symmetric axis) inside of the colon lumen; (2) building a radial varying cylinder which is inscribed within the inner wall of the colon lumen. Several methods have been presented for centerline extraction for medical imaging [6]. Combined with the Fast Marching technique [19], an energy minimization formula is given as follows [20],

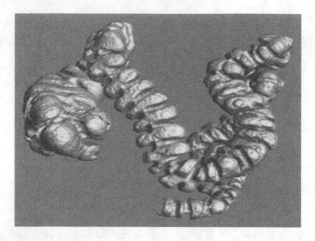

Fig. 2 SL mesh after marching cube

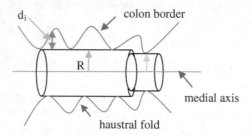

Fig. 3 The cylinder model

$$E_{medial-Axis}(C) = \int_{0=C^{-1}(p_0)}^{L=C^{-1}(p_1)} F(C(s))ds \qquad (2)$$

where F(x) is a scalar filed, and C=C(s) (s being arc length)is the path(traced from two points p_0 and p_1) along which we look for the centerline. What we need to do is to minimize E. In this study, we employed a method to solve a nonlinear hyperbolic partial differential equation [21]. Let $|\nabla T(x)|=F(x)$, then we have,

$$T(x) = \min_{C \in \Gamma(p_0,x)} \left(\int_{0=C^{-1}(p_0)}^{\bar{s}=C^{-1}(x)} F(C(s))ds \right) \qquad (3)$$

where $\Gamma(p_0, x)$ is the set of all paths from p_0 to x. Since the scalar field $T(x)$ represents weighted geodesic distance to point p_0, the weighted geodesic paths are orthogonal to level sets of $T(x)$. Once the field of weighted geodesic distances has been found, the weighted geodesic path of interest is calculated by constructing a path from p_1 oriented as $\nabla T(x)$ in every point. The medial axis is a set of points, $C(\tilde{p})$, $\tilde{p} \in \Omega, \Omega$ stands for the colon object. Then the shortest distance between the points

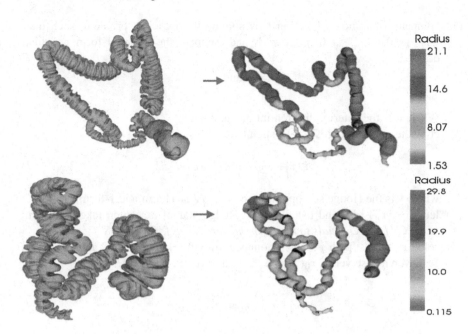

Radius
21.1

14.6

8.07

1.53

Radius
29.8

19.9

10.0

0.115

Fig. 4 Illustration of the cylinder of colon (Different colors stands for the varying distance)

on the medial axis and the vertices on the colon surface ($\partial\Omega$) can be expressed as,

$$\{r_i = \min(d_i)|d_i = \sqrt{(\tilde{p}_j - v_i)^2}, \tilde{p}_j \in C(\tilde{p}), v_i \in \partial\Omega\} \tag{4}$$

where r_i is the radius of the cylinder model. The colon inscribed cylinders are shown in Fig. 4.

This constructed cylinder has its' own surface ($\partial\Omega''$), the Euclidean distance between the vertices on the colon surface and the surface of the cylinder will be further calculated as follows,

$$\{D_i = \min(z_i)|z_i = \sqrt{(v_i - l_j)^2}, v_i \in \partial\Omega, l_j \in \partial\Omega''\} \tag{5}$$

where l_j is a vertex on the $\partial\Omega''$, and v_i is a vertex on the $\partial\Omega$. The set of D, named distance map, will be further introduced in the following flattening process.

2.4 Improved Flattening Map Model of Colon Wall

In recent years, a number of methods have been proposed to map the colon surface to a plane or a sphere [5]. For best eliminating the limitations brought by 2D flattening image, we introduce the 2.5D flatten techniques. Given a colon surface Ω (as shown in Fig. 2), with boundaries γ_0, γ_1, then we can,

(1) compute a Harmonic function f by solving the Dirichlet problem, such that: $|\Delta f \equiv 0, |f|_{\gamma_0} \equiv 0, f|_{\gamma_1} \equiv 1$, and compute the closed 1-form τ, which denotes:

$$d\tau = 0, \text{ and } \int_{\gamma_0} \tau = 1 \tag{6}$$

Where d is the exterior differential operator;
(2) compute a function g: $\Omega \rightarrow R$, such that,

$$\xi(\tau + dg) = 0, \text{ and } \xi = {}^*d^* \tag{7}$$

where * is the Hodge star operator and $\tau + dg$ is a harmonic 1-form;
(3) let $\omega = \tau + dg$, and calculate the Hodge star of ω, which takes the form ${}^*\omega = Cdf$ and C equals to the harmonic energy of f: $C = \int_\Omega |\nabla f|^2$;
(4) select a shortest path γ, which connects γ_0 with γ_1, and slice Ω along γ to get $\overline{\Omega}$. Given a base vertex $v_0(v_0 \in \overline{\Omega})$, for any vertex $v(v \in \overline{\Omega})$,

$$\varphi(v) = \int_{v_0}^{v} \omega + \sqrt{-1} * \omega, \tag{8}$$

where φ is the flattening mapping and $\omega + {}^*\omega\sqrt{-1}$ is Holomorphic 1-form.
Along the integration path which may be chosen arbitrarily on $\overline{\Omega}$, we finally got the mapping between any vertex (x,y,z) in 3D and the new vertex(x', y', z')(**Note**: z' equals to the corresponding D_i for vertex (x, y, z)) .

3 Applications

The new 2.5D flattening model can be applied to the following: (1) To improve navigation experience in VC,(2) to help detecting haustral folds on the colon wall, and (3) to find out the taniae coli line of colon (see Fig. 5). In this paper, we performed two applications: haustral folds detection& segmentation and TC finding.

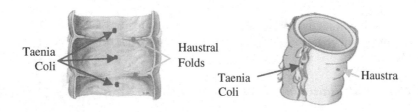

Fig. 5 Illustration of Teniae coli, haustra and haustral folds

3.1 Haustral Folds Detection and Segmentation

In previously reported literature, most research methods in the field mainly focused on fold detection, rather than fold segmentation. For example, in [3, 22], folds were detected by thresholding the curvatures in three-dimensional (3D) colon representation, while in [4], the detection task was fulfilled by using a Gabor filter on a 2D unfolded colon representation. A local elevation histogram (LEH) method is proposed for the colonic folds detection or segmentation. The main idea is divided into four steps: (1) dividing the whole flattening colon along the colon wall into several equal parts (experimentally the length of each unit equals to one eighth of the narrowest haustral fold); (2) calculating the average distribution of the elevation(local elevation) along the direction parallel to the walking direction of colon wall; (3) checking the minimum elevation value (MinEv): if (MinEv) is more than the maximum elevation value (MaxEv), then neglect the current part, else if (4) using the split lines (red bold, as shown in Fig. 8) to determine which part belongs to haustral folds. It should be noted the threshold (the value on the L) is manually obtained by creating a cutting plane.

However, mean curvature flow can be exploited in fold segmentation process. As shown in Fig. 7, the peak and the valley can both be determined by the high (positive) or low (negative) curvatures.

3.2 Teniae Coli Extraction for Colon

Teniae coli (TC) are three approximately 8-mm-wide longitudinal smooth muscle bands in the colon wall. In previously reported literature, approaches for extraction the Teniae coli can be categorized into two groups, manual drawing and automatic extraction [3, 4, 22]. As far as the automatic approaches to be concerned, most of previous researchers suggested to use curvature filter or Gabor filter [4] for surface analysis to get the TC lines on the colon. However, TC usually appears to be with the middle height between the haustra and the haustral folds. Fortunately, this phenomenon can be apparently found in the proposed 2.5D flattened colon (as shown in Fig. 6). Therefore, extracting the TC lines equals to finding the shortest geodesic path on the 2.5 D flattened map. The new algorithm for TC extraction is described in Algorithm 2. In this algorithm, we can randomly pick up three arbitrary vertices along the top edge of the colon flattened mesh (as shown in Fig. 9). Equally, we will choose four vertices at the other end of the colon.

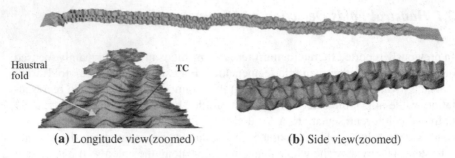

Haustral fold

TC

(a) Longitude view(zoomed)   **(b)** Side view(zoomed)

Fig. 6 The 2.5D effects of the flattening model

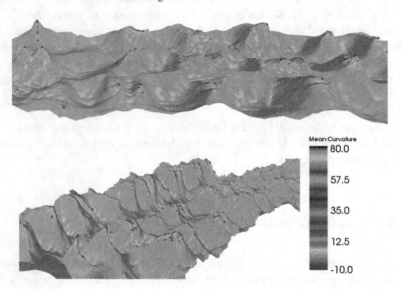

Mean Curvature

80.0

57.5

35.0

12.5

-10.0

Fig. 7 The 2.5D effects of the mean curvature(*blue* points indicate the higher curvature, *yellow* points indicate the relative lower curvature, the rest are *green*)

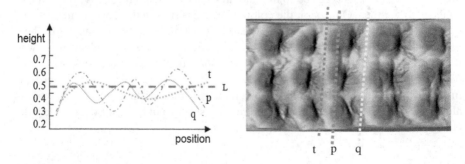

Fig. 8 The smoothed profile lines and an experimental result of colon fold segmentation

---
Algorithm 1 *Shortest path finding for the TC extraction*

Given the flattened colon mesh graph
  S := empty sequence
  u := target
for each vertex v in Graph:
  dist[v] := infinity ;   //Initializations
  path[v] := Flag of Undefined ; // Previous node in optimal path
  end for   // from source
dist[source] := 0 ;   // Geodesic distance from source to source
Ω := the set of all nodes in Graph ;   // All nodes in the graph
while Ω is not empty: // The main loop
    // Start node in first case on the top of stack
    while path[u] is Flag of Defined: // Construct the
    shortest path with a stack S
        insert u at the beginning of S   // Push the vertex into the
        stack
        u := path[u]   // Traverse from target to source
    end while ;
    remove u from Ω ; //--improve the efficiency
    for each neighbor v of u: // where v has not yet been removed from Ω.
      alt := dist[u] + dist_between(u, v) ;
        if alt < dist[v]:
          dist[v] := alt ;
          path[v] := u ;
        end if
    end for
  end while
  return S;

3.3 Evaluation

To evaluate the haustral folds segmentation and the TC extraction, ground truth was established from 15 patient scans by experts' drawing of the fold boundaries. According to the suggestions from experts, a haustral fold would be detected if more than 50 % of its area has been detected. As we mentioned before, the maximum elevation value (MEV) needs to be manually determined according to the position of the cutting plane. Experimental result shows that the different case requires different MEV to get the good performance (as shown in Fig. 10). In practice, the MEV ranges from 0.28 to 0.51 for the 2.5D flattening results. Figure 10 illustrates the sensitivity which varies with the MEV. The average detection true positive (TP) rate is 93.2 %, which is slightly better than that reported in [8]. While for the TC extraction, in most cases, the new approach can draw the approximate TC lines for the colon wall with no much deviation.

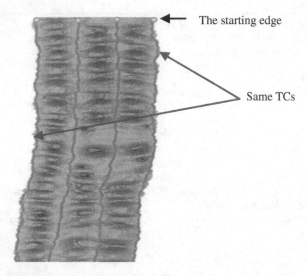

Fig. 9 The result of TC extraction

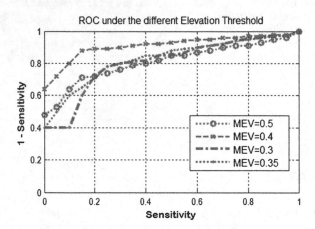

Fig. 10 The ROC under different MEV

4 Conclusion

A novel colon flattening model based on 2.5D approach for describing the structure of colon wall is presented in this work. The algorithm uses a novel method which detects the accurate PV layer of colon via a MAP-EM partial segmentation algorithm. A level set based shrinkage method is then applied to generate a much better approximated mucosa surface representing the inner surface of the colon wall. We further present a new approach to describe the undulation of the inner colon wall. An elevation distance map is introduced to depict the neighborhood characteristics of the inner colon wall. Coupling with the conformal flattening model, the new proposed approach provides a new vision for colon analysis in CTC studies. We have shown the effectiveness of our algorithm on segmenting haustral folds segmentation and detecting three TCs. This newly proposed model shall further advance computer aided detection and diagnosis in CTC studies.

Acknowledgments This work was partially supported by the NIH/NCI under Grant #CA143111, #CA082402, and the PSC-CUNY award #65230-00 43.

References

1. American Cancer Society (2012) Cancer facts & figures 2012. American Cancer Sciety, Atlanta
2. Eddy D (1990) Screening for colorectal cancer. Ann Intern Med 113:373–384
3. Lamy J, Summers R (2007) Teniae coli detection from colon surface: extraction of anatomical markers for virtual colonos-copy. In: LNCS, vol 4841, pp 199–207
4. Wei Z, Yao J, Wang S, Summers R (2010) Teniae coli extraction in human colon for computed tomographic colonography images. In: Proceedings of the MICCAI 2010 workshop: virtual colonoscopy & abdominal imaging, pp 135–140. Beijing, China
5. Hong W, Gu X, Qiu F, Jin M, Kaufman A (2006) Conformal virtual colon flattening In: Proceedings of the 2006 ACM symposium on solid and physical modeling, pp 85–93
6. Wan M, Liang Z, Ke Q, Hong L, Bitter I, Kaufman A (2002) Automatic centerline extraction for virtual colonoscopy. IEEE Trans Med Imaging 21:1450–1460
7. Zeng W, Marino J, Gu X, Kaufman A (2010) Conformal geometry based supine and prone colon registration. In: Medical image computing and computer-assisted intervention (MICCAI) virtual colonoscopy, workshop, pp 149–154
8. Zhu H, Barish M, Pickhardt P, Liang Z (2013) Haustral fold segmentation with curvature-guided level set evolution. IEEE Trans Biomed Eng 60(2):321–331
9. Paik DS, Beaulieu CF, Jeffrey RB Jr, Karadi CA, Napel S (2000) Visualization modes for CT colonography using cylindrical and planar map projections. J Comput Assist Tomogr 24(2):179–188
10. Haker S, Angenent S, Kikinis R (2000) Nondistorting flattening maps and the 3D visualization of colon CT images. IEEE Trans Med Imaging 19:665–670
11. Bartrolf A, Wegenkittl R, Konig A, Groller E (2001) Nonlinear virtual colon unfolding. In: Proceedings of IEEE visualization, pp 411–418
12. Bartroli AV, Wegenkittl R, Koumlnig A, Groumlller E (2001) Nonlinear virtual colon unfolding. In: Proceedings of IEEE Visualization, pp 411–418
13. Wang Z, Li B, Liang Z (2005) Feature-based texture display for detection of polyps on flattened colon volume. In: Proceedings of the 2005 IEEE engineering in medicine and biology 27th annual conference Shanghai, China, 1–4 Sept 2005
14. Jin M, Kim J, Luo F, Gu XD (2008) Discrete surface ricci flow. IEEE Trans Visual Comput Graphics 14(5):1030–1043
15. Zeng W, Marino J, Chaitanya GK, Gu X, Kaufman A (2010) Supine and prone colon registration using quasi-conformal mapping. IEEE Trans Vis Comput Graphics 16:1348–1357
16. Yao J, Chowdhury AS, Aman J, Summers RM (2010) Reversible projection technique for colon unfolding. IEEE Trans Biomed Eng 57(12):2861–2869
17. Liang Z, Yang F, Wax M, Li J, You J, Kaufman A, Hong L, Li H, Viswambharan A (1997) Inclusion of a priori information in segmentation of colon lumen for 3D virtual colonoscopy. In: Conference record of IEEE nuclear science symposium-medical imaging conference, Albuquerque, NM
18. Sethian JA (1999) Level set methods and fast marching methods: evolving interfaces in computational geometry, fluid mechanics, computer vision, and materials science, 2nd edn. Cambridge University Press, Cambridge

19. Sethian JA (1996) A fast marching level set method for monotonically advancing fronts. Proc Nat Acad Sci 93:1591–1595
20. Deschamps T, Cohen LD (2001) Fast extraction of minimal paths in 3D images and appli-cation to virtual endoscopy. Med Image Anal 4:281–299
21. Antiga L (2003) Patient-specific modeling of geometry and blood flow in large arteries. PhD thesis, Politecnico di Milano
22. Huang A, Roy DA, Summers RM, Franaszek M, Petrick N, Choi JR, Pickhardt PJ (2007) Teniae coli-based circumfe-rential localization system for CT colonography: feasability study. Radiology 243(2):551–560
23. Williams D, Grimm S, Coto E, Roudsari A, Hatzakis H (2008) Olumetric curved planar refor-mation for virtual endoscopy. IEEE Trans Visual Comput Graphics 14(1):109–119

Biomechanical Simulation of Lung Deformation from One CT Scan

Feng Li and Fatih Porikli

Abstract We present a biomechanical model based simulation method for examining the patient lung deformation induced by respiratory motion, given only one CT scan input. We model the lung stress-strain behavior using a sophisticated hyperelastic model, and solve the lung deformation problem through finite element (FE) analysis. We introduce robust algorithms to segment out the diaphragm control points and spine regions to carefully define the boundary conditions and loads. Experimental results through comparing with the manually labeled landmark points in real patient 4DCT data demonstrate that our lung deformation simulator is accurate.

1 Introduction

The use of four-dimensional computed tomography (4DCT) has becoming a common practice in radiation therapy, especially for treating tumors in thoracic areas. There are two alternative methods for 4DCT acquisition, namely retrospective slice sorting and prospective sinogram selection. No matter which method is used, the prolonged acquisition time results in a considerably increased radiation dose. For example, the radiation dose of a standard 4DCT scan is about 6 times of that of a typical helical CT scan and 500 times of a chest X-ray. Moreover, 4DCT acquisition cannot be applied to determine the tumor position in-situ. These facts have become a major concern in the clinical application of 4DCT, motivating development of advanced 4DCT simulators.

Towards this goal, various approaches have been proposed to model lung inflation/deflation. The first category of methods discretize the soft tissues (and bones) into masses (nodes) and connect them using springs and dampers (edges) based on mass-

F. Li (✉) · F. Porikli (✉)
Mitsubishi Electric Research Laboratories, Cambridge, MA 02139, USA
e-mail: feng.d.li@gmail.com

F. Porikli
e-mail: fatih.porikli@gmail.com

J. M. R. S. Tavares et al. (eds.), *Bio-Imaging and Visualization for Patient-Customized Simulations*, Lecture Notes in Computational Vision and Biomechanics 13, DOI: 10.1007/978-3-319-03590-1_2, © Springer International Publishing Switzerland 2014

spring-damper system and CT scan values for spline-based MCAT phantoms [15], augmented reality based medical visualization [14], respiration animation [22], tumor motion modeling [20], and etc. Conventionally, they apply affine transformations to the control points to simulate respiratory motion. Lungs and body outline are linked to the surrounding ribs, such that they would have the synchronized expansion and contraction [15]. These approaches can only provide approximate deformations.

The second category of methods use hyperelastic models to describe the non-linear stress-strain behavior of the lung. The straightforward way to simulate lung deformation between two breathing phases (T_i, T_{i+1}) is to use the lung shape at T_{i+1} as the contact/constraint surface and deform the lung at T_i based on the predefined mechanical properties of lung [8, 17]. In this case, a negative pressure load on the lung surface is applied and Finite Element (FE) analysis is used to deform tissues [21]. The lung will expand according to the negative pressure and slide against the contact surface to imitate the pleural fluid mechanism [3]. This pressure can be estimated from the patient's pleural pressure versus lung volume curve, which in turn are measured from pulmonary compliance test [19]. Along this line, patient-specific biomechanical parameters on the modeling process for FE analysis using 4DCT data are learned in [18]. A deformable image registration of lungs study to find the optimum sliding characteristics and material compressibility using 4DCT data is presented in [1].

Besides lung deformation, the displacements of rib cage and diaphragm are also very important to design a realistic 4DCT simulator. Didier et al. [4] assume the rib cage motion is a rigid transformation and use finite helical axis method to simulate the kinematic behavior of the rib cage. They develop this method into a chest wall model [5] relating the ribs motion to thorax-outer surface motion for lung simulation. Saadé et al. [13] build a simple diaphragm model consisting of central tendon and peripheral muscular fibre. They apply cranio-caudal (CC) forces on each node of the muscular fibre to mimic the diaphragm contraction and use Gauchy-Green deformation tensor to describe the lung deformation. Hostettler et al. [9] consider *internal organs* inside the rib cage as a convex balloon and estimate internal deformation field directly through interpolation of the skin marker motions.

Patient-customized deformation approaches often assume a 4DCT of the patient is already available. We note that simulating deformations without any 4DCT has many challenges as lung motion changes considerably depending on health condition (with or without cancer), breathing pattern (abdomen vs. chest wall), age and many other factors. Nevertheless, 4DCT simulation without any prior (e.g. 4DCT of the same patient) is useful for developing treatment strategy in image-guided radiotherapy and generating controlled data to design and evaluate X-ray video based medical solutions.

In this paper, we present a biomechanical model based thoracic 4DCT simulation method that can faithfully simulate the deformation of lung and nearby organs for the whole breathing cycle. Our method takes only one CT scan as input, and defines the loads on the rib cage and the diaphragm to constrain the lung deformation. This differentiates our method from conventional continuum mechanics based algorithms. In the extended version of this paper, we also simulate the passive mass-spring model

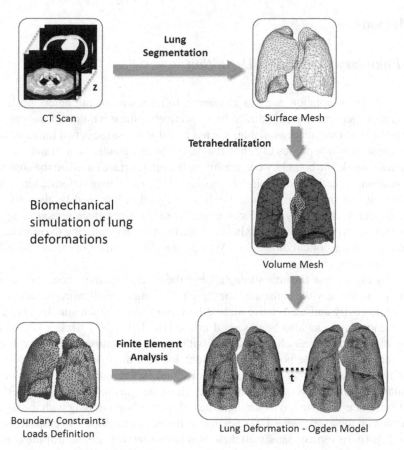

Fig. 1 Processing pipeline of our biomechanical simulation of lung deformations from one CT scan. The tetrahedra on the cutting plane of the volume mesh are colored in *purple*. *Red* points indicate imposed automatic boundary constraints

based deformation of abdominal organs due to lung inflation/deflation. Conversion from density to mass assumptions for mass-spring model are supported by clinical data. To evaluate the accuracy of our simulator, we perform both qualitative image visual examination and quantitative comparison on expert annotated lung interior point pairs between multiple breathing phases, and demonstrate that our biomechanical model based simulation is very accurate. Figure 1 shows the processing pipeline of our 4DCT simulator based on biomechanical model.

2 Methods

2.1 Boundary Constraints Definition

For simplicity of notation, we use x, y and z to represent lateral, anterioposterior (AP), and superoinferior (SI) direction respectively. Since we do not assume we have a 4DCT of the patient available, it is not possible to use the actual lung surfaces of different breathing phases to define the deformation boundary constraints.

Instead, we define boundary constraints on the lung surface based on the anatomy and function of the human respiratory system [16] for the lung deformation. First, considering that the upper lobes of the lung are well constrained by the ribs, the displacement vectors (x, y and z components) of the tip surface region of upper lobes are fixed to avoid a pure translation of the lung when simulating the diaphragm contracting on the bottom of the lung. We take the clinical study in [6] as a basis for these constraints.

During inspiration, the lung sliding against the rib cage mainly occurs in the posterior/spine region, while in the anterior region, the lung expands with the increasing of thoracic cavity and the relative sliding between them is much smaller [11, 23]. This phenomenon can also be observed in the DIR-Lab 4DCT dataset [2], which is one of the most recent clinical studies with expert annotations for this problem. Therefore, we define the boundary conditions for both the front and the back parts of the lung surface in order to simulate the different sliding actions. As shown in the boundary constraints box of Fig. 1, our system fixes the z displacement for all surface mesh vertices marked in red to simulate the coherent motion of lung with the thorax expansion on the axial plane. The selection of the vertices is based on empirical evidence [2]. These vertices satisfy all these heuristics that they are on/near the convex hull of the lung surface, around the lateral sides of the middle and lower lobes, and have small ($<20°$) normal variations.

To simulate the pleural sliding in the spine region, our simulator automatically locates the lung surface vertices in the vicinity of the thoracic vertebrae, and fixes the x and y displacements of these points as the third boundary constraint. Notice that our goal is to find surface vertices close to the spine, therefore we design a simple Gaussian curve fitting algorithm to locate these points instead of adopting a complicated thoracic vertebrae segmentation approach. The idea is to fit a set of Gaussian curves such that the area cut out by each curve is maximized. This provides a good global approximation to the spine shape and the constraint points can be accurately located. For simplicity, considering a sample 2D axial view, our algorithm maximizes the light blue region A covered by the blue Gaussian curve $f(x) = ae^{-\frac{(x-b)^2}{2c^2}}$, as shown in Fig. 2a.

We formulate it as a constrained multi-variable optimization problem as:

$$\max_{a,b,c} \sum_{x=x_{min}}^{x_{max}} f(x), \quad \text{s.t. } f(x) - g(x) \leq 0, \forall x \in [x_{min}, x_{max}], \tag{1}$$

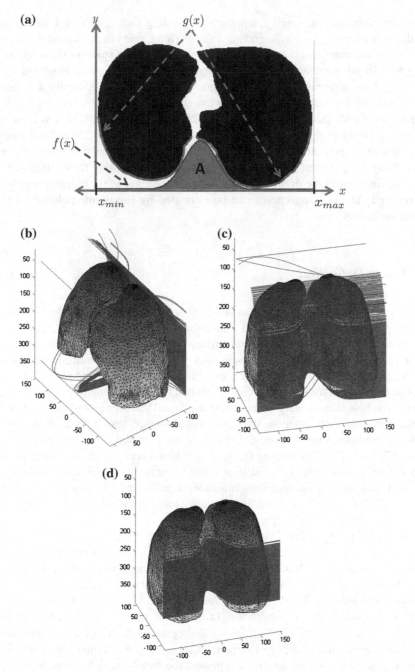

Fig. 2 Gaussian curve fitting for spine region estimation: **a** 2D Gaussian curve fitting on a CT slice, **b** and **c** the different views of our 3D curve fitting results, and **d** final curve fitting result after outliers are removed

where the parameter a, b and c represent the scaling factor, expected value, and standard variance of $f(x)$, x_{min} and x_{max} are the lung limits in the lateral direction, and $g(x)$ is the upper limit for $f(x)$ and is the minimum y value of the lung slice at each x. In our simulator, this constrained optimization problem is solved very efficiently by a sequential quadratic programming method, specifically active-set algorithm, which computes a quasi-Newton approximation to the Hessian of the Lagrangian at each iteration. We extend this 2D algorithm to the 3D CT volume by simply applying this algorithm slice by slice, as can be seen in Fig. 2b and c. Outliers occur in the top and bottom of the lung where $g(x)$ is only partial constraints for the curve fitting. Our simulator removes these outliers by computing their difference to the mean Gaussian curve of the set, therefore correct fittings of the thoracic vertebrae are retained. The missing curves can be estimated by linear interpolation of the remaining curves.

2.2 Loads Definition

Since we are given one input CT scan and there is no bounding surface at the second breathing phase, we design an extra traction applied on the diaphragm area of the lung besides the negative intra-pleural surface pressure. The pressure force inflates the lung in all directions during inspiration, while the traction allows additional displacement in z direction to mimic the diaphragm contraction and pleural sliding.

Note that the pressure force can be well defined from the simulator input, therefore we focus on how to accurately locate the points (faces) that are close to the diaphragm for the definition of the traction. We model this as a graph search problem and solve it by our modified shortest closed-path algorithm. Our simulator first computes a dense 3D point cloud by finding the lung voxels at every (x, y) location with the largest z value, as shown in Fig. 3c, then converts the point cloud into a weight map, Fig. 3d, based on the local geometry information, and finally locates the diaphragm points (Fig. 4f) through our modified shortest closed-path algorithm. The left and right lower lobe are treated separately.

Weight Map Definition: We consider the 3D point cloud as an 2D image with intensity value from the z value of the corresponding point, and run the local Line Direction Discrepancy (LDD) computation on this image to generate the weight map W. Thus our weight map computation can also be viewed as a special type of image filtering. As shown in Fig. 3a, for each line $d_i(x, y)$ of a block centering at (x, y), we build up two sub-lines $d_i^1(x, y)$ and $d_i^2(x, y)$ from (p_i^3, p_i^2, p_i^1) and (p_i^3, p_i^4, p_i^5) respectively, $(i = 1, \ldots, 4)$, and compute the LDD as the minimum intersection angle of the four sub-line pairs. Alternatively, we compute the maximum of the cosine value of these angles to represent the weight, which can be efficiently calculated through dot product as

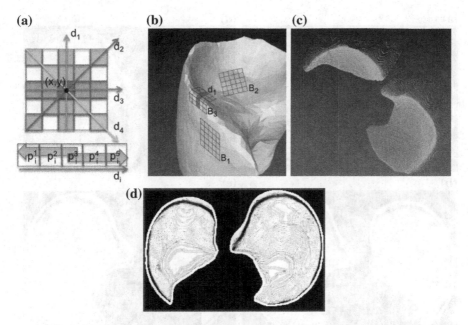

Fig. 3 Weight map calculation for diaphragm point segmentation. **a** The line direction definition of our LDD measure. **b** Sample blocks on the lung surface to illustrate our weight calculation algorithm. The orange region d_1 of B_1 has the highest LDD value out of the three sample blocks. **d** The weight map corresponding to the input point cloud (**c**)

$$W(\mathbf{p}) = \max_{i=1,\ldots,4} \{\frac{d_i^1 \cdot d_i^2}{\| d_i^1 \| \cdot \| d_i^2 \|}\}, \tag{2}$$

where $\mathbf{p}$ represents pixel position (x, y), and the block size is set as 5×5 for simplicity. Intuitively, regions with high curvature would high/positive LDD value, for example, d_1 of B_3 in Fig. 3b, while flat regions would have low/negative LDD values, for instance, B_1 and B_2.

Diaphragm Point Segmentation: Notice that all outliers locate at the boundary of the weight map, thus we formulate the diaphragm point segmentation as a shortest closed-path (SCP) problem, which finds a optimal cut along the boundary that separates the diaphragm points from the outliers. To build the graph for SCP, we choose 4 neighborhood connection and set the edge weight $E_{\mathbf{pq}}$ as $W(\mathbf{q})$. Therefore, $E_{\mathbf{pq}}$ and $E_{\mathbf{qp}}$ may have different weights. Instead of using the entire weight map to build the graph, we mask out the inner region through morphological operations and limit the optimal cut (red curve) between the inner $\partial \Omega_2$ and outer boundary $\partial \Omega_1$ (blur curves), as shown in Fig. 4a. If we directly adopt the idea from [10] to design the SCP algorithm, some interior regions would be inevitably cut out to favor the lowest cost, as shown in Fig. 4b and c.

To solve this problem, we first sample the outer boundary $\partial \Omega_1$ every 10 points and find their corresponding points (in terms of Euclidean distance) on the inter

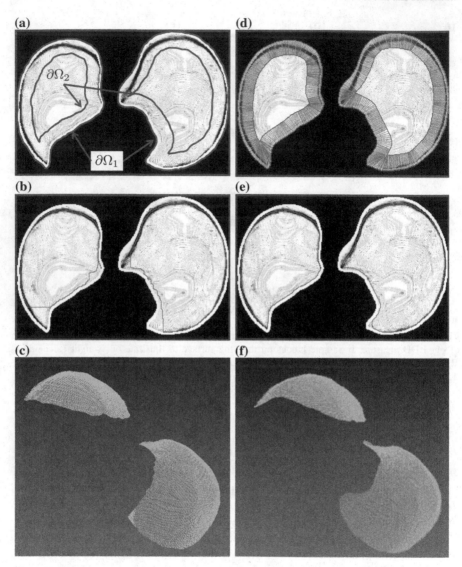

Fig. 4 Diaphragm point segmentation. **a** Masked out the inner region: the inner $\partial\Omega_2$ and outer boundary $\partial\Omega_1$ (*blue curves*). **b** The optimal cut by conventional SCP algorithm (in *red*). **c** The estimated diaphragm points. Our new SCP algorithm unbends the ring regions in **d** into ribbon belts, and can accurately segment out the diaphragm points for traction definition in (**e**) and (**f**)

boundary $\partial\Omega_2$, as the green lines shown in Fig. 4d. For the rest points on $\partial\Omega_1$, we compute their matches on $\partial\Omega_2$ (purple lines) through linearly interpolation of the previous matches (green lines), such that there are no crossing matches (lines) and correct ordering could be maintained. In this way, we can unbend the ring region between $\partial\Omega_1$ and $\partial\Omega_2$ into a ribbon belt by aligning up all the purple and green lines in order, and set the length of the ribbon as the length of $\partial\Omega_1$ and the width as the shortest distance between $\partial\Omega_1$ and $\partial\Omega_2$. We then build up a new adjacency matrix/graph from the ribbon for the SCP algorithm. As we can see from Fig. 4e and f, this would give us the accurate diaphragm points for the traction definition.

2.3 Finite Element Simulation

The final step for biomechanical simulation of lung deformation is to define the material property of the lung and apply FE analysis. We assume the lung tissue is homogeneous, isotropic, and use the first-order Ogden model [12] to describe its non-linear strain energy density function as

$$W(\lambda_1, \lambda_2, \lambda_3, J) = \frac{\mu_1}{\alpha_1}(\lambda_1^{\alpha_1} + \lambda_2^{\alpha_1} + \lambda_3^{\alpha_1} - 3) + \frac{K}{2}(\ln J)^2, \qquad (3)$$

where $\lambda_{1,2,3}$ are the deviatoric principal stretches, μ_1 and α_1 are material constants, J is the Jacobian of the lung deformation, and K is the bulk modulus chosen sufficiently high to satisfy near-incompressibility. Here, we choose the Ogden parameters from [7] for all our experiments, $\mu_1 = 0.0329$, and $\alpha_1 = 6.82$.

Next, we combine all the information (meshes, loads, and boundaries) defined in the previous sections into a single script file and directly run a FE solver to simulate the lung deformation. We integrate the open-source FEBio [7] into our simulator as the FE solver, and a lung deformation example is shown in Fig. 5.

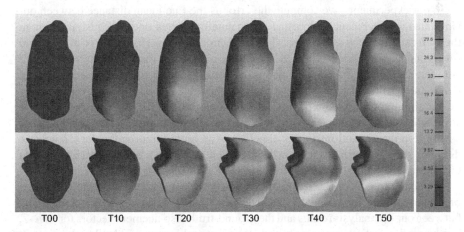

Fig. 5 Finite element analysis of a left lung deformation during inspiration. The *top row* displays the posterior view and the *bottom row* shows the inferior view. Color shows the degree of displacement with red denoting maximum displacement

Table 1 Mean error (and standard deviation) of the deformed lungs measured in 3D space and its x, y, and z components in mm

Case ID	CT Dims	Our Results	Hostettler et al.[9]
Case7	$512 \times 512 \times 136$	3.79 (1.80)	5.31 (3.35)
Case8	$512 \times 512 \times 128$	6.15 (3.31)	10.81 (4.69)
Case9	$512 \times 512 \times 128$	3.17 (1.37)	5.86 (1.83)
Case10	$512 \times 512 \times 120$	4.37 (2.95)	6.93 (2.86)

This table demonstrates that our biomechanical simulation algorithm for lung deformation is accurate and performs better than [9] on tested DIR-Lab 4DCT datasets [2]

3 Results and Discussion

Figure 5 shows an example of FE analysis of a left lung deformation during inspiration. The simulation results resemble the real 4DCT lung deformation with the maximum displacement occurring in the posterior region along the SI direction. The results also demonstrate realistic lung inflating effect due to the negative surface pressure, which can be better viewed in the second row of the figure. In our FE analysis, we define the simulation time for the inspiration phase is 2 seconds with step size $\Delta t = 0.1$, pressure force -0.02 and traction 0.005. For other parameters, for example, convergence tolerance, we use the default values in the FEBio solver.

To demonstrate the accuracy of our FE simulation, we evaluate our simulator on the DIR-Lab 4DCT dataset [2]. We use the cases with 512×512 slice resolution. Each test case has 300 manually labeled landmark points between T_{ex} and T_{in}. For instance, *case-7*, which has an average landmark displacement of 11.59 ± 7.87 (standard deviation) mm, and the observer error of 0.81 ± 1.32 mm. Detailed specifications of the dataset can be found at http://www.dir-lab.com.

In our experiments, we compute the error as the Euclidean distance between our simulated displacement vectors and the manually labeled ones. We also implement the deformation filed estimation algorithm proposed by Hostettler et al. [9], and set its model parameters using the ground-truth marker displacement vectors. We compare its simulation results with ours in Table 1, and the detailed distributions of simulation errors for *case-7* in Fig. 6. From the table, we can see that the accuracy of our simulator improves roughly 40 % compared with [9]. The reasons why our simulator has larger errors in z direction are twofold. First, human lung generally has strong respiratory motions in this direction. And more importantly, the CT volume data has stronger artifacts and lower resolution in z than x and y, considering that the spatial resolution of tested CT data is $0.97 \times 0.97 \times 2.5$ mm.

We compute the error as the Euclidean distance between the simulated displacement vectors and the manually labeled ones. In Fig. 7, we show the comparison between our FE analysis results and the ground-truth displacement vectors for *case-7*. For better illustration, we only show the left lung, which has 153 landmark points. It can be seen that our simulator generates accurate results in the lower posterior region where the nodal displacement is mostly prominent. We observe that our simulation results have some angular difference with the manually labeled data in the upper

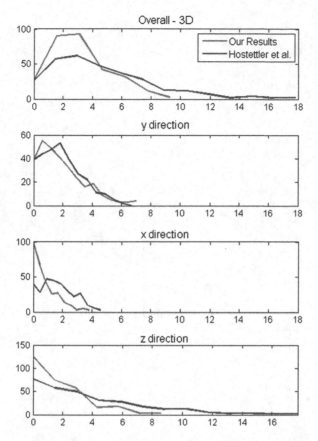

Fig. 6 Mean error distributions of our simulation results and Hostettler et al. [9] for overall 3D, and in x, y, and z directions for *case7*. Horizontal axes are the error magnitudes in *mm*. As visible, our simulator has more accurate estimation

anterior region. That is partially due to lack of other prior force definitions for these elements in the simulator as it only uses the negative surface pressure. Besides, it is possible that the manually identified landmark points contain large errors since nodal displacement in this region is less than or around the z spatial resolution of the CT dataset.

We implement the deformation filed estimation algorithm proposed by Hostettler et al. [9], and set its model parameters using the ground-truth marker displacement vectors. We compare its simulation results with ours in Table 1. From the table, we can see that the accuracy of our simulator improves roughly 40 % compared with [9]. As indicated by [2], these test cases have very different patient lung shapes, tumor sizes and locations, and breathing mechanisms. A simple interpolation between axial lung envelopes adopted by Hostettler et al. [9] inevitably generates large errors while our algorithm adapts to different patients, thus achieves comparably more accurate results as shown in Table 1.

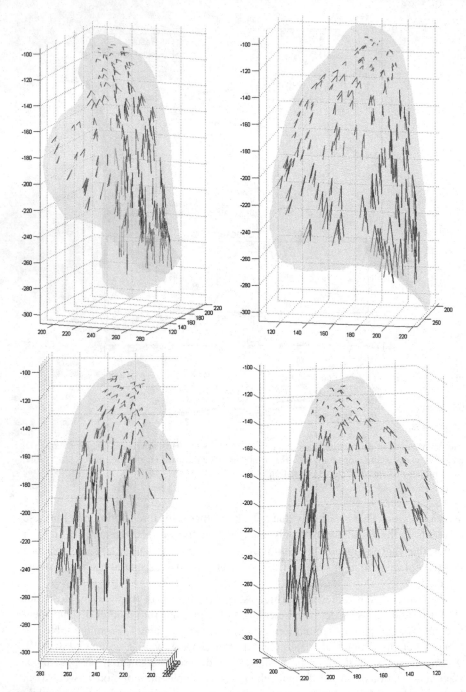

Fig. 7 Comparison between our simulated displacement vectors and ground-truth data at manually identified landmark positions for *case-7*. The *blue lines* represent the ground truth displacement of the landmark points between T_{ex} and T_{in}, while the *red lines* represent our simulation results

Our algorithm is a patient-customized lung deformation simulator. By providing more sophisticated constraints, the simulation quality will improve further. For instance, the patient lung surface in *case-8* is heavily curved in the back/posterior region, thus including extra constraints to maintain this curved lung shape may make the simulation more precise.

4 Conclusions

We have present a biomechanical model based lung simulation method for examining the patient lung deformation induced by respiration given only one CT scan input. We model the lung stress-strain behavior using a hyperelastic model, and simulate the lung deformation by defining accurate boundary constraints and loads. Extensive analysis and comparisons with the manually labeled DIR-Lab dataset demonstrate that our lung deformation results are accurate.

References

1. Al-Mayah A, Moseley J, Velec M, Brock K (2009) Sliding characteristic and material compressibility of human lung: parametric and verification. Med Phys 36(10):4625–4633
2. Castillo R, Castillo E, Guerra R, Johnson V, McPhail T, Garg A, Guerrero T (2009) A framework for evaluation of deformable image registration spatial accuracy using large landmark point sets. Phys Med Biol 54:1849
3. DiAngelo E, Loring S, Gioia M, Pecchiari M, Moscheni C (2004) Friction and lubrication of pleural tissues. Respir Physiol Neurobiol 142(1):55–68
4. Didier A, Villard P, Bayle J, Beuve M, Shariat B (2007) Breathing thorax simulation based on pleura physiology and rib kinematics. In: IEEE international conference on medical information visualisation-biomedical visualisation
5. Didier A, Villard P, Saadé J, Moreau J, Beuve M, Shariat B (2009) A chest wall model based on rib kinematics. In: IEEE international conference on visualisation
6. Ehrhardt J, Werner R, Frenzel T, Lu W, Low D, Handels H (2007) Analysis of free breathing motion using artifact reduced 4DCT image data. In: SPIE medical imaging conference
7. Ellis B, Ateshian G, Weiss J (2012) FEBio: finite elements for biomechanics. J Biomech Eng 134(1):5–11
8. Eom J, Shi C, Xu X, De S (2009) Modeling respiratory motion for cancer radiation therapy based on patient-specific 4DCT data. In: MICCAI
9. Hostettler A, Nicolau S, Forest C, Soler L, Remond Y (2006) Real time simulation of organ motions induced by breathing: first evaluation on patient data. In: Biomedical simulation conference
10. Jia J, Sun J, Tang C, Shum H (2006) Drag-and-drop pasting. In: ACM SIGGRAPH conference
11. Norman W (1999) The anatomy lesson. Georgetown University, Washington
12. Ogden R (1972) Large deformation isotropic elasticity-on the correlation of theory and experiment for incompressible rubberlike solids. Proc R Soc Lond Ser A Math Phys Sci 326(1567):565–584
13. Saadé J, Didier A, Villard P, Buttin R, Moreau J, Beuve M, Shariat B (2010) A preliminary study for a biomechanical model of the respiratory system. In: International conference on computer vision theory and applications

14. Santhanam A, Fidopiastis C, Hamza-Lup F, Rolland J, Imielinska C (2004) Physically-based deformation of high-resolution 3d lung models for augmented reality based medical visualization. In: Medical image computing and computer aided intervention, AMI-ARCS, pp 21–32
15. Segars W, Lalush D, Tsui B (2001) Modeling respiratory mechanics in the MCAT and spline-based MCAT phantoms. IEEE Trans Nucl Sci 48(1):89–97
16. Vidiâc B, Suarez F (1984) Photographic atlas of the human body. CV Mosby (St. Louis)
17. Villard P, Beuve M, Shariat B, Baudet V, Jaillet F (2005) Simulation of lung behaviour with finite elements: influence of biomechanical parameters. In: IEEE international conference on medical information visualisation-biomedical visualisation, 2005
18. Werner R, Ehrhardt J, Schmidt R, Handels H (2009) Patient-specific finite element modeling of respiratory lung motion using 4DCT image data. Med Phys 36(5):1500–1511
19. West J (2008) Respiratory physiology: the essentials. Lippincott Williams and Wilkins, Philadelphia
20. Wilson P, Meyer J (2010) A spring-dashpot system for modelling lung tumour motion in radiotherapy. Comput Math Methods Med 11(1):13–26
21. Zhang T, Orton N, Mackie T, Paliwal B (2004) Technical note: a novel boundary condition using contact elements for finite element based deformable image registration. Med Phys 31(9):2412–2415
22. Zordan V, Celly B, Chiu B, DiLorenzo P (2006) Breathe easy: model and control of simulated respiration for animation. Graph Models 68(2):113–132
23. Zuckerman S (1963) A new system of anatomy. Oxford University Press, London

2D–3D Registration: A Step Towards Image-Guided Ankle Fusion

Ahmed Shalaby, Aly Farag, Eslam Mostafa and Todd Hockenbury

Abstract In this paper, we introduce a new framework for registering pre-operative 3D volumetric data to intra-operative 2D images. We are particularly interested in examining the problem of aligning CT volumes to corresponding X-ray images. Our objective is to apply the 2D-3D registration in the field of orthopedics, specifically on ankle fusion surgery. Our framework adopts the shear-warp factorization (SWF) method to generate synthetic 2D images from the given 3D volume. Also, the alignment score is determined based on two novel similarity measures; the exponential correlation (EC) and the pixel-based individual entropy correlation coefficient (IECC). Our framework has been tested on 22 clinical CT datasets. We used different methods to evaluate registration quality of our system. Evaluation results confirm the degree of accuracy and robustness of our proposed framework.

Keywords Shear-warp factorization · Optimization · Registration · CT · X-ray

A. Shalaby (✉) · A. Farag · E. Mostafa
Computer Vision and Image Processing Laboratory, University of Louisville,
Louisville, KY, USA
e-mail: ahmed.shalaby@louisville.edu

A. Farag
e-mail: aly.farag@louisville.edu

E. Mostafa
e-mail: eamost01@louisville.edu

T. Hockenbury
Department of Orthopedic Surgery, University of Louisville, Louisville, KY, USA
e-mail: todd.hockenbury@insightbb.com

J. M. R. S. Tavares et al. (eds.), *Bio-Imaging and Visualization for Patient-Customized Simulations*, Lecture Notes in Computational Vision and Biomechanics 13, DOI: 10.1007/978-3-319-03590-1_3, © Springer International Publishing Switzerland 2014

1 Introduction

The registration of pre-operative 3D volumetric images to intra-operative 2D images provides an important way for relating the patient position and medical instrument location. In applications from orthopedics [1, 2] to neurosurgery [3], it has a great value in maintaining up-to-date information about changes due to surgical intervention [4].

The widely used 3D image modalities such as Magnetic Resonance Imaging (MRI), Computed Tomography (CT) and Positron Emission Tomography (PET) contain high resolution information about the imaged part of the human body. All these modalities can be greatly used for pre-operative procedure planning or evaluating an intervention post-operatively. However, the main drawback of these images is not completely reflecting the surgical situation, since they are static. In some applications it is important to use intra-operative images to follow the changes caused by the procedure or to visualize the location of a tool [4]. In the operating room (OR), 2D images are more suitable for recording details about the current state. X-ray images are good examples of image modalities used for this purpose. Unfortunately, 2D images lack significant information that is present in the 3D modalities. So that, in order to relate between the OR 2D images and the detailed 3D model, experts need to mentally combine the information from the pre-operative and intra-operative images which is a very tough task. Therefore, it is useful to find a way to automate that procedure and making it reliable. The fusion of pre-operative and intra-operative images will be meaningful if the components are properly aligned in space. To achieve this it is necessary to determine their relative position and orientation. The procedure that identifies a geometrical transformation that aligns two datasets is called registration [4]. There are several approaches that can perform this task. Unfortunately, all of these techniques work on images of the same dimensionality, i.e. inputs are either 2D or 3D. But in our case, we need to align images with different dimensionality and combine the information from high-resolution pre-operative datasets with the updated intra-procedural images. Additionally, as the registration results are expected during the medical procedure, the computation time would also be constrained [4].

In this paper, we introduce a simple framework for 2D-3D registration of human ankle using X-Ray and CT Images. Our system consists of three main steps: (1) Projection of the pre-operative 3D volume to generate a synthetic 2D image, (2) Similarity measurement to quantify the quality of the alignment between the generated image and the reference (intra-operative) image, and (3) Optimization process to modify and refine current estimates of the problem parameters in a way that the similarity score is maximized. In many registration systems, the quality of alignment is scored by objective functions. Common registration methods can be grouped into two major categories based upon the nature of the similarity measure to which they apply: they can be classified as feature or intensity-based. Feature-based methods rely on the identification of natural landmarks in the input images in order to determine the best alignment. It is necessary to segment the most significant features in both of the input images and the matching criterion is then optimized with respect to them.

Intensity-based methods operate on the pixel intensities directly. They calculate various statistics using the intensity values of the inputs which are compared in the images to be aligned. According to literatures, intensity-based similarity measures are more suitable for 2D-3D applications [2]. They suggested many objective functions that can be used in matching X-ray and CT images. For example: normalized cross-correlation [2], pattern intensity [5], normalized mutual information (NMI) [6, 7], gradient correlation and gradient difference [2]. The rest of this paper is organized as follows: Sect. 2 talks about the long-term application of our work. Section 3 discusses the background of methods used in our experiment. Section 4 explains the experiments, and evaluates the accuracy of our results. Finally, conclusions are drawn in Sect. 5.

2 Applications

The majority of the medical applications for the proposed kind of registration have emerged in the field of radiology. Alignment information is important in planning, guidance and treatment procedures. This kind of work is crucial for the field of orthopedics and neuroradiology. It can be used in the following areas: Cranio-Catheter procedures, Metastatic Bone Cancer, Hip Re-placement, and Spine Procedures [3]. Our collaborators are interested in applying the 2D-3D registration in the field of orthopedics. The major project is image-guided ankle fusion surgery. The long-term goal of this work is to apply this technique to ankle fusion surgery to determine the proper size and orientation of the screws which are used for fusing the bones together. In addition, we try to localize the best bone region to fix these screws. An ankle fusion is a surgical operation usually done when an ankle joint becomes worn out and painful. The most common cause of this pain is an ankle fracture. After a serious fracture, the joint may wear out and become painful. For example, a joint that is out of balance after it heals from a fracture can wear out faster than normal. As shown in Fig. 1, an ankle fusion removes the surfaces of the ankle joint and allows the tibia to grow together, or fuse, with the talus [8]. The cut ends of the tibia and talus are brought together and held in place with three screws. Based on the intra-operative X-ray images, the doctor decides the size, the length, and the orientation of these screws. Our ultimate goal is to enhance the quality of the surgical procedure in terms of time and accuracy, and would greatly reduce the need for repeated surgeries; thus, saving the patients time, expense, and trauma.

We are proposing to create an image-guided tool that would allow the screws selected to be the proper length, and the angle selected to be the optimum angle, to fuse tibia to the talus, but not allow the screws to protrude through the talus into the Subtalar joint, as shown Fig. 2. The first step of that tool is the 2D-3D registration process. The process, in short, is aligning a 3D model based on pre-operative CT scans to corresponding 2D X-ray image acquired in the operation room (OR).

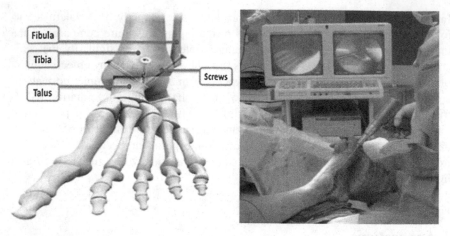

Fig. 1 Ankle fusion surgery

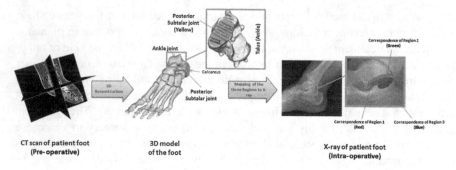

Fig. 2 Components of the image-guided ankle/foot surgery

3 Methods

In our application, we focus on fusing CT and X-ray images. One of the key challenges when studying the 2D-3D registration problem is the need for an appropriate way to compare input datasets that are of different dimensionalities. One of the most common approaches is to simulate one of the modalities given the other dataset and an estimate about their relative spatial relation-ship, so that the images can be compared in the same space. Then a transformation T estimate can be updated to maximize the alignment according to some similarity measure. Most existing applications simulate 2D images from the 3D volume. Its more feasible to follow this approach. Simulated projection images that are to model the production of X-ray acquisitions from 3D volumetric CT are called Digitally Reconstructed Radiographs (DRRs). Figure 3 describes the main components of our framework. We first apply 3D translations t_x, t_y, t_z and rotations $\theta_x, \theta_y, \theta_z$ to the CT volume. Using the CT volume, we perform projection to generate the DRR. We define the projected image

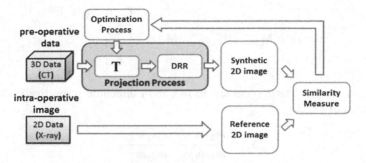

Fig. 3 The block diagram of 2D-3D registration process

(DRR) as the floating image and the X-ray image as the reference image. After the projection step, we have to identify a similarity measure that can quantify the quality of the alignment between the images and defining a procedure to modify and refine current estimates of the transformation parameters (rotation and translation) in a way that the similarity score is optimized. In other words, provided that we have a suitable similarity function, the best alignment parameters can be located with the help of an optimization procedure. More details about our framework will be discussed in the following subsections.

3.1 Projection Process

We use a shear-warp factorization (SWF) method to generate synthetic 2D images from a given 3D CT volume (DRR images). It is one of the latest techniques of volume rendering [3]. In this method, a viewing transformation is applied to simplify the projection processing which is the mapping of world coordinates of the object into a virtual camera coordinates. The algorithm uses a principal viewing axis to choose a set of CT voxel slices to be resampled and composited. It also determines the order of the slices along the front-to-back direction of the image volume [9]. Let M_{view} be a 4×4 affine viewing transformation matrix that transforms points from the object space to the image space. As shown in Fig. 4, M_{view} can be factorized as $M_{view}=M_{warp} M_{shear}$. As discussed in [4], the shear transformation matrix M_{shear} can be described as:

$$M_{Shear} = \begin{bmatrix} 1 & 0 & s_x & 0 \\ 0 & 1 & s_y & 0 \\ 0 & 0 & 1 & 0 \\ 0 & 0 & 0 & 1 \end{bmatrix}. \tag{1}$$

The second factor of the viewing matrix describes how to warp the intermediate image into the final image. So, we can get:

$$M_{warp} = M_{view} . M_{Shear}^{-1} = M_{view} \cdot \begin{bmatrix} 1 & 0 & -s_x & 0 \\ 0 & 1 & -s_y & 0 \\ 0 & 0 & 1 & 0 \\ 0 & 0 & 0 & 1 \end{bmatrix}, \tag{2}$$

where s_x, s_y are the shearing coefficients in x and y directions respectively, and $m_{i,j}$ are elements of M_{view}, as:

$$S_x = \frac{m_{22} m_{13} - m_{12} m_{23}}{m_{11} m_{22} - m_{21} m_{12}}, \tag{3}$$

$$S_y = \frac{m_{11} m_{23} - m_{21} m_{13}}{m_{11} m_{22} - m_{21} m_{12}}, \tag{4}$$

where $m_{i,j}$ are elements of M_{view}. Figure 4b shows samples for projected 2D images using SWF approach with different viewing parameters (i.e. different t_x, t_y, t_z, θ_x, θ_y, θ_z). The average elapsed time required to generate a DRR image (based on SWF) is 3.920.45 s. More details about SWF and volume rendering techniques can be found in [1–5, 9, 10].

3.2 Similarity Measure

In our framework, two novel image similarity measures are adopted from [11] and [12]. The first one is called exponential correlation (EC). The other is called pixel-based individual entropy correlation coefficient (IECC). Both are used as the similarity measure between the DRR images and the reference X-ray image in order to evaluate the current quality of alignment.

3.2.1 Exponential Correlation (EC)

Given that the real X-ray image is the reference image (R) and the DRR image is the floating image (F), their EC value can be calculated using the following equation:

$$EC(R, F) = E\left[\left(e^{F(\mathbf{x}) - \overline{F}} - 1 \right) \left(e^{R(\mathbf{x}) - \overline{R}} - 1 \right) \right], \tag{5}$$

where $\mathbf{x}$ stands for the coordinates vector of the image, the vector $\mathbf{x}$ is defined on the set D_X defined as $F \cup R$ [11], and $E[.]$ denotes the expectation operator over the D_X. $\overline{F}$ and $\overline{R}$ represent the mean of intensity values of images F and R respectively. When two images are geometrically aligned, EC value is maximized.

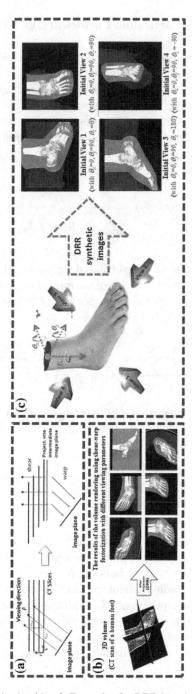

Fig. 4 **a** Shear-warp factorization idea. **b** Examples for DRR based on SWF. **c** The initialization scenarios

3.2.2 Individual Entropy Correlation Coefficient (IECC)

In this type of similarity measures, we deal with the images R and F as two random variables. A 1D histogram is constructed for each image. It shows the distribution of the pixel values. Since these values vary over a wide range, they were rescaled into $N = 64$ bins. A 2D histogram $h(r,f)$ is obtained from the pair of floating image and reference image. Each entry in this histogram represents the number of times intensity r in image R coincides with intensity f in the other image F. The probability distribution of this 2D histogram values is obtained from $h(r,f)$. It is called the joint probability distribution and can be expressed as:

$$p(r_i, f_j) = \frac{h(r_i, f_j)}{\sum\limits_{i=1}^{N} \sum\limits_{j=1}^{N} h(r_i, f_j)} \qquad (6)$$

As discussed in [12], the pixel-based IECC depends on $p(r_i, f_j)$. It represents the ratio between the pixel-based component of the mutual information between the two images, and the sum of the pixel-based components of the two marginal entropies of each image. So, IECC is expressed as:

$$\text{IECC}(R, F) = \sum_{i=1}^{N} \sum_{j=1}^{N} \frac{p(r_i, f_j) \log_2 \left(\frac{p(r_i, f_j)}{p(r_i) p(f_j)} \right)}{p(r_i) \log_2 p(r_i) + p(f_j) \log_2 p(f_j)}, \qquad (7)$$

where $p(r_i)$ and $p(f_j)$ are the marginal probability distribution of each image. When two images are geometrically aligned, IECC value is maximized. For more details, see [12].

3.3 Optimization Process

Provided that we have a suitable similarity function, the best alignment parameters can be estimated with the help of an optimization process. The optimization process aims to maximize the similarity score between images. There are two major classes of optimization approaches: non-gradient and gradient methods. The first class might be easier to implement as it requires only the evaluation of the objective function and no additional computations to derive the consecutive search directions. However, the second could potentially be much faster as its search is guided towards the maximum. For simplicity, we use NelderMead method (one of non-gradient methods) in our system [1].

(a)   (b)   (c)   (d)   (e)

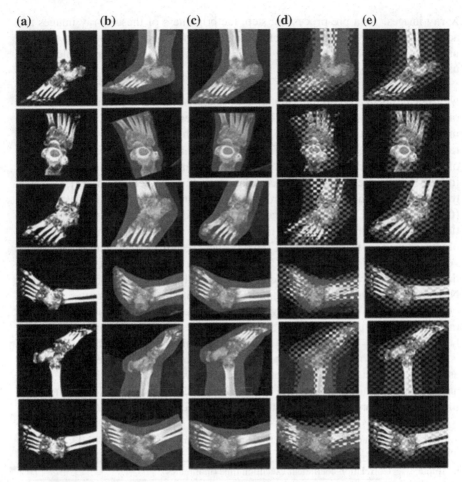

Fig. 5 2D-3D Registration results for different examples with different views for one of our clinical datasets using IECC as a similarity measure: **a** is the reference image (represents the intra-operative X-ray generated by ray-casting algorithm) **b** is the initial floating (synthetic) image, generated by SWF algorithm **c** is the final floating image after registration, **d** is checkerboard representation before registration and **e** after registration

4 Experimental Results

In this paper, we apply our framework on clinical CT ankle datasets. The goal is to register these pre-operative CT data to intra-procedural 2D images. The clinical datasets were scanned at 120 kV with 2.5 mm, 1.33 mm, 0.67 mm, or 0.42 mm slice thicknesses. We tested our algorithm on 1500 CT slices which are obtained from 15 different patients. Regarding the intra-operative 2D images, we use the shear-warp factorization method to generate ground truth X-ray images with different viewing transformations (i.e. known $t_x, t_y, t_z, \theta_x, \theta_y, \theta_z$) that represent the intra-operative

X-ray images. As a pre-processing step, the brightness of these X-ray images are adjusted to roughly segment the soft tissues from the ankle bones (see Fig. 5a). We use these images to test the quality of our system. All algorithms are implemented using Matlab 7.[1]

We used a variety of methods to measure the accuracy of our framework. First, we used the checkerboard representation to visually evaluate the registration quality of our framework (see Fig. 5d, e. In these examples, we use IECC as a similarity measure. Having a closer look at Fig. 5e, it shows that the registration is very accurate, since the two parts coming from different images have no transition. Edges of the foot bone are connected along the squares in all parts of the checkerboard image. Second, we computed the correlation coefficient (defined in [13]) between the image R and the image F before and after registration using NMI (described in [6]), EC, and IECC for different examples with different viewing parameters. Additionally, we measure the execution time required for each example (in minutes). The obtained results are summarized in Table 1. These results indicate that: For the interventional applications, although EC based framework is not the most accurate, it has the advantage of reducing the execution time by almost two third as compared to NMI and IECC. On the other hand, if the accuracy is sought, IECC outperforms the other two systems with comparative execution time to NMI approach. Finally, the mean error—and its standard deviation SD—of the estimated registration parameters $t_x, t_y, t_z, \theta_x, \theta_y, \theta_z$ using NMI, EC and IECC are summarized in Table 2. This error is the average absolute difference between the ground truth parameters and the final estimated parameters after registration of a given view for all CT datasets. Again, and according to these results, the accuracy of the IECC framework is higher than the systems that are based on the other similarity measures; NMI and EC.

Table 1 Correlation coefficient of our 2D-3D registration framework using NMI, EC and IECC for different views

Example	Correlation coefficient/execution time (in minutes)			
	Before registration	After registration (NMI)	After registration (EC)	After registration (IECC)
View 1	0.6297	0.8234/2.9	0.8174/1.1	0.9974/2.7
View 2	0.6102	0.8511/2.7	0.8741/0.9	0.9851/2.5
View 3	0.5162	0.8923/3.0	0.8886/1.2	0.9904/3.1
View 4	0.5716	0.8959/3.2	0.8896/0.9	0.9934/2.9
View 5	0.5234	0.8738/3.6	0.8835/1.3	0.9884/3.2
View 6	0.6453	0.9003/2.3	0.8921/0.7	0.9986/2.0
View 7	0.5015	0.812/3.3	0.8236/1.5	0.9158/3.2
View 8	0.4325	0.7887/4.2	0.7912/2.1	0.8368/4.0
View 9	0.6235	0.8325/2.8	0.8553/0.9	0.9684/2.6
View 10	0.5108	0.8351/3.2	0.8125/1.3	0.9213/2.9

The red values represent the execution time (in minutes)

---

[1] All algorithms are run on a PC with a 2 GHz Core i7 Quad processor with 8GB RAM.

Table 2 Mean registration error and SD of the estimated parameters

Parameters		t_x(mm)	t_y(mm)	t_z(mm)	$\theta_x(deg)$	$\theta_y(deg)$	$\theta_z(deg)$
Error	NMI	1.1 ± 0.91	1.2 ± 0.89	1.4 ± 0.98	1.0 ± 0.77	1.2 ± 0.87	0.6 ± 0.62
	EC	1.3 ± 0.86	0.9 ± 0.79	1.6 ± 0.99	0.9 ± 0.78	1.3 ± 1.01	0.7 ± 0.48
	IECC	0.9 ± 0.52	0.8 ± 0.41	1.1 ± 0.69	0.7 ± 0.36	0.9 ± 0.41	0.4 ± 0.29

5 Conclusions and Future Work

In this paper, we introduced a simple framework for registering pre-operative 3D volumetric data to intra-operative 2D images in the field of orthopedics, specifically on ankle surgery. Our framework was implemented based on SWF rendering techniques with EC or Individual Entropy Correlation Coefficient (IECC) as new similarity measures for the 2D-3D registration process. It was tested on different clinical CT scans of human ankle and foot. Experiments demonstrated that our EC-based framework is fast and per-forms almost as good as NMI which is compatible with the time limitation of the interventional applications. From the accuracy point of view, the IECC-based framework is the most accurate system with comparative execution time to NMI-based system. Our proposed approach can be considered as a step towards a robust image-guided surgical station for ankle fusion surgery. Future directions are geared towards formulating a new objective function and implementing an advanced optimization technique to expand our work. We are also aiming to apply the 2D-3D registration on real X-ray image (Not synthetic images). This requires a dataset of X-ray and CT images for the same patient. Also, it is very important to validate our framework on a large number of datasets (up to 100 scans). We are also aiming to speed up our framework by adopting modern graphics processing units (GPUs) for direct volume rendering.

References

1. Bifulco P, Cesarelli M, Allen R, Romano M, Fratini A, Pasquariello G (2010) 2D–3D Registration of CT vertebra volume to fluoroscopy projection: a calibration model assessment. EURASIP J Adv Sign Proces 1–8
2. Penney GP, Weese J, Little JA, Desmedt P, Hill DLG, Hawkes DJ (1998) A comparison of similarity measures for use in 2D–3D medical image registration. IEEE Trans Med Imaging 17(4):586–595
3. Markelj P, Tomazevic D, Likar B, Pernus F (2010) A review of 3D/2D registration methods for image-guided interventions. Med Image Anal 16(3):642–661
4. Zollei L (2001) 2D-3D rigid-body registration of x-ray fluoroscopy and CT images. Master Thesis, Massachusetts Institute of Technology, Cambridge
5. Weese J, Buzug TM, Lorenz C, Fassnacht C (1997) An approach to 2D/3D registration of a vertebra in 2D x-ray fluoroscopies with 3D, CVRMed/MRCAS'97, France, 19–22 March 1997
6. Viola P, Wells W (1997) Alignment by maximization of mutual information. Int J Comput Vision 24(2):137–154
7. Pluim PW, Maintz JBA, Viergever MA (2000) Image registration by maximization of combined mutual information and gradient information, Proc MICCAI 1935:452–461

8. http://www.myanklereplacement.com/
9. Chen X, Gilkeson RC, Feia B (2007) Automatic 3D-to-2D registration for CT and dual-energy digital radiography for calcification detection. Med Phys 34(12):4934–4943
10. Weese J, Penney GP, Desmedt P, Hill DLG, Hawkes DJ (1997) Voxel-based 2-D/3-D registration of fluoroscopy images and CT scans for image-guided surgery. IEEE Trans Info Technol Biomed 1(4):284–293
11. Kalinic H, Loncaric S, Bijnens B (2011) A novel image similarity measure for image registration. 7th International Symposium on Image and Signal Processing and Analysis (ISPA), 2011
12. Itou T, Shinohara H, Sakaguchi K, Hashimoto T, Yokoi T, Souma T (2011) Multimodal image registration using IECC as the similarity measure. Med Phys 38(2):1103–1115
13. Maintz J, Viergever M (1998) A survey of medical image registration, Med Image Anal 2(1):1–36

A Graph Based Methodology for Volumetric Left Ventricle Segmentation

S. P. Dakua, J. Abi Nahed and A. Al-Ansari

Abstract Clinician-friendly methods for cardiac image segmentation in clinical practice remain a tough challenge. Despite increased image quality including medical imaging, image segmentation continues to represent a major bottleneck in practical applications due to noise and lack of contrast. Larger standard deviation in segmentation accuracy may be expected for automatic methods when the input dataset is varied; also at some instances the radiologists find them hard in case any correction is desired. In this context, this paper presents a semi-automatic algorithm that uses anisotropic diffusion for smoothing the image and enhancing the edges followed by a new graph cut method, AnnularCut, for 3D left ventricle segmentation from some pre-selected MR slices. The main contribution, in this work, is a new formulation for preventing the cellular automation method to leak into surrounding areas of similar intensity. Another contribution is the use of level sets for segmenting the slices automatically between the preselected slices segmented by the cellular automaton. Both qualitative and quantitative evaluation performed on York and MICCAI Grand Challenge workshop database of MR images reflect the potential of the proposed method.

Keywords Cellular automata · Graph cut · Segmentation · MR

S. P. Dakua (✉) · J. Abi Nahed
Qatar Science and Technology Park \ QRSC, Qatar Foundation, Deha, Qatar
e-mail: sdakua@qstp.org.qa

J. Abi Nahed
e-mail: jabinahed@qstp.org.qa

A. Al-Ansari
Hamad Medical Corporation, Qatar Foundation, Deha, Qatar
e-mail: aalansari1@hmc.org.qa

J. M. R. S. Tavares et al. (eds.), *Bio-Imaging and Visualization for Patient-Customized Simulations*, Lecture Notes in Computational Vision and Biomechanics 13, DOI: 10.1007/978-3-319-03590-1_4, © Springer International Publishing Switzerland 2014

1 Introduction

Magnetic resonance imaging (MRI) is a noninvasive modality for imaging the heart, that helps physicians to properly diagnose. Some of its advantages viz. (1) low ionizing radiation, (2) ability to provide maximum information for diagnosis by a single test and (3) less operator dependence, keep it ahead of other imaging modalities like X-ray, CT scan and PET etc. Precise measurement of left ventricle (LV) shape being the basis for surgery planning, an accurate segmentation always remains as an essential requirement. A rich tradition of work in image segmentation has focused on the establishment of appropriate image (object) models; in fact, the literature on segmentation techniques is huge ([8, 14, 19] for example).

1.1 MR Image Segmentation Techniques

If we consider manual segmentation, it is not only a tedious and time consuming process but also an inaccurate one. Segmentation by experts is variable up to 20 % [41], it is therefore desirable to use algorithms that are accurate and require little user interaction such as active contour. This basically includes parametric active contour (or snake) and geometric active contour (or level set). Snake is an automatic procedure with little user interaction. Snake model [18, 37] is reliable in poor resolution images but the topology is to be known in advance. Moreover, the initial contour needs to be initialized near to the object boundary. The accuracy of its segmentation depends on the parameters defined by the user. When more splitting and merging occur then the problem arises in the adaptability of the algorithm. Level set methods [11, 23, 28] that have been extensively used in medical image segmentation overcome some of the limitations. Although level set methods gained tremendous popularity, still some problems like computational complexity, re-initialization [20, 29] of the zero level set exist. In the early level set methods, the computation is carried out on the entire domain making the computation slow. Narrow band level set methods [2] restrict the computation to a narrow band around the zero level set, but it does not reduce the computational cost to a reasonable limit. Similarly, expectation maximization (EM) [38] algorithm has the ability to estimate the parameters of different classes but fails to utilize the strong spatial correlation between neighboring pixels. Stabilized inverse diffusion equations [16], based on a simple spring-mass model suffers from well defining the force function. Integration of fuzzy logic with data mining techniques has become one of the key constituents of soft computing in handling the challenges posed by massive collections of natural data. The fuzzy clustering algorithms allow the clusters to grow into their natural shapes. Fuzzy c-means clustering is similar to k-means clustering in many ways but incorporates fuzzy set concepts of partial membership and forms overlapping clusters to support it. Such a method [33] is reported to be applicable to any dimensional representation and at any resolution level of an image series. The main drawback of this method is from the restriction that the sum of membership values of a data point in all the clusters must be one and this tends to give high membership values for the outlier points. So the algorithm has difficulty in handling outlier points. Secondly, the membership of a data point in a cluster depends directly on its membership values in other cluster centers and this sometimes happens to produce unrealistic results. Thirdly, its inability to calculate the membership value if the distance of a data point is zero.

Normalized cut [17], suffers from high noise present in medical images. Active contours without edges [7] is useful in automatic detection of interior contours but to discriminate regions, mean intensities are to be different. Atlas registration [21] is a recognized paradigm for the automatic segmentation of normal CMR images. The method uses non-rigid registration to elastically deform a cardiac atlas built automatically from different normal subjects. Unfortunately, atlas-based segmentation has been of limited use in presence of large space-occupying lesions. There also many model based segmentation techniques [10] but, one limitation of the model-based segmentation is that the model might converge to the wrong boundaries. Segmentation with ratio cut [35] does not produce correct segmentations for boundaries aligned with image edges. The algorithm relies on the shape of the object, while the approach in [39] sometimes causes over segmentation. The mixture of fuzzy and EM algorithm [30] is useful for automatic LV segmentation but the complexity in validation is more; the EM algorithm has to be stopped before a deteriorating "checkerboard effect" [15] shows up.

Stochastic active contour scheme (STACS) [32] for automatic image segmentation is designed to overcome the normal problems with low contrast and turbulent blood flow. The difficulty lies in the modeling, which requires the prior knowledge of the heart for a better assessment of the object boundary. Michael et al. [25] extract the myocardium of the LV using a level-set segmentation process. Again the level set method requires manual specification of the free parameters, at the cost of some error. Sum and Paul have proposed an approach [36] for vessel extraction using a level set based active contour. But it is less capable in handling bifurcations and the sensitivity to imaging artifacts, producing discontinuities of the coronary vessels. Its accuracy can only be improved by incorporating a priori information on vessel anatomy. A fast and semiautomatic algorithm proposed in [12] is based on random walk approach. It does not carry any assumption/condition, but the selection of initial seeds on various labels is a tough task in slow intensity varying CMR images.

1.2 Motivation

A much larger standard deviation of the final scores can be observed for automatic methods; on the other hand, a semi-automatic (with reasonable interactions) method is more suitable because of being able to guide the resulting contour as per the desire of the clinician [14]. Without doubt, graph-based methods have advanced our understanding of image segmentation and have successfully been employed since sometime without heavy reliance on explicitly learned/encoded priors. Intelligent scissors is a boundary-based interactive method, that computes minimum-cost path between user-specified boundary points [26]. However, this is unable to integrate any regional bias naturally, which is overcome by the Graph Cut method as follows. Graph Cut [6] is a combinatorial optimization technique; the globally optimal pixel labeling can be efficiently computed by maxflow/min-cut algorithms. Grab Cut [34] extends Graph Cut by introducing iterative segmentation scheme. There are also other graph based image segmentation methods in the literature, such as Random Walk [1] and the list continues. However, the performance of most of the graph-based methods typically rely on the weighting function [17] and it is a tough task to define this, especially, for medical images. This is because medical images have their own unique properties. In many cases, the objects to be segmented are very different in their structure and appearance from the objects that are common in photo editing. Probably that is why much research effort is being applied to develop efficient segmentation methods in this domain. This paper presents a clinician friendly semi-automatic algorithm that is based on graph theory for left ventricle (LV) segmentation.

2 Methods and Materials

As a pre-processing step, the algorithm utilizes the basic anisotropic diffusion filtering to enhance the edges in the image where different objects are minutely distinct and then the method for segmentation follows subsequently. The proposed method for segmentation resembles graph cut, where the seeds for foreground (FG) and background (BG) are defined by the user in a polygon manner (shaped like a ring), hence the name *AnnularCut*; it provides an efficient mean of selecting the region of interest.

2.1 Background

Cellular automaton (CA) [40] is an innovative concept for pixel labeling from an initialized curve C_{object}. A (bi-directional, deterministic) CA is a triplet $A = (S, N, \delta)$, where S is an non-empty state set, N is the neighborhood system, and $\delta : S^N \rightarrow S$ is the local transition function (rule). This function defines the rule of calculating the cells state at $t + 1$ time step, given the states of the neighborhood cells at previous time step t. The cell state S_p is actually a triplet $(I_p, \theta_p, \mathbf{C}_p)$—the label I_p of the current cell, strength of the current cell θ_p, and cell feature vector $\mathbf{C}_p$, defined by the image; $\theta_p \in [0, 1]$. The meaning of the triplet remains same with the change in subscript (say p to q), it is only a matter of change of nodes. When user starts the segmentation by specifying the segmentation seeds, the seeded labels are set accordingly, while their strength is set to the seed strength value; this sets the initial state of the process. At iteration $t + 1$ cell labels I_p^{t+1} and strengths θ_p^{t+1} are updated, for example, if

$g\left(\left\|\mathbf{C}_p - \mathbf{C}_q\right\|_2\right) \cdot \theta_q^t > \theta_p^t$ then $I_p^{t+1} = I_q^t$ and $\theta_p^{t+1} = g\left(\left\|\mathbf{C}_p - \mathbf{C}_q\right\|_2\right) \cdot \theta_q^t$; g is a monotonous decreasing function. The calculation continues until automaton converges to a stable configuration, where cell states seize to change.

There are certain problems with traditional CA when applied to real medical images; for example some CA methods, in the presence of noise, produce directed percolation [9] and noise is inherent to the process of medical data acquisition, therefore naive application of CA usually leads to pseudo results (as shown in Sect. 4). Furthermore, the intensity values of the LV tissue at certain regions are often similar to that of adjacent structures. The above two problems combining together exacerbate above described convergence yielding poor results. We therefore propose to use dynamic cellular automation (DCA) [9] that considers the minimal energy between two cells along with the image features and their distance to calculate g and strength θ mitigating convergence problem and improving the performance.

2.2 DCA for Image Segmentation

Continuing with the above discussion, let $\{x_1, \ldots, x_n\}$ be a set of binary variables (object and background), then the energy sum of (up to two) variables can be written as: $E(x_1, \ldots, x_n) = \sum_i E^i(x_i) + \sum_{i<j} E^{i,j}(x_i, x_j)$. The goal is to find an equivalent g, in terms of energy,

$$E\left(\mathbf{C}_p\right) = \sum_{p \in P} D_p\left(\mathbf{C}_p\right) + \sum_{p,q \in \aleph} V_{p,q}\left(\mathbf{C}_p, \mathbf{C}_q\right) - \frac{\mathbf{C}_p}{\max \|\mathbf{C}\|} \tag{1}$$

where $\aleph \subset P \times P$ is a neighborhood (4 in this case) system on pixels. The first term in the energy function is typically called the data term, D, consisting of the total penalty in assigning each pixel a label. The second term of the function is typically called the smoothness term, V, Kolmogorov's terminology. The cells grow on the seeded region, but when the object cells are minutely differed from the neighboring cells with respect to intensity (as in the case of LV MR image) the probability of final contour to cross the actual boundary becomes higher. Therefore, some boundary conditions are required to prevent the contour from crossing the actual boundary. For this, we have introduced another polygon (a set of seed points) surrounding the object of interest. The similar operation (as in the above seeded region) is performed in this seeded ($C_{background}$) region too.

During CA operation, at each iteration, new curves C_{object} and $C_{background}$ are determined and subsequently, the following energy minimization is determined. Once both snakes (one for the object and one for the background) are optimized, all cellular automata operations stop, otherwise, the procedure continues further iteratively. At each iteration, the new curve energy is calculated as:

$$E(C) = \int_0^1 \left[\alpha(s) \left| \frac{\partial v}{\partial s} \right|^2 + \beta(s) \left| \frac{\partial^2 v}{\partial s^2} \right|^2 - |\nabla u_0(v(s))|^2 \right] \tag{2}$$

where α, β and γ are real-valued coefficients which balance the different contributions to the snake energy. s denotes the curvilinear abscissa and $v(s)$ the point of co-ordinates $x(s)$, $y(s)$ on the curve and u_0 is the image. The curve is assumed to be closed, annulling the derivative of this functional with respect to the contour C leads to the following Euler-Lagrange equation

$$\alpha \kappa(s) \vec{N} + \beta \frac{\partial^4 v}{\partial s^4} - \gamma \nabla \left[|\nabla u_0(v(s))|^2 \right] = 0 \tag{3}$$

When a curve is parameterized by the curvilinear abscissa, we get $\frac{\partial^2 v}{\partial s^2} = \kappa(s) \vec{N}$, where $\kappa(s)$ is the local curvature and $\vec{N}$ the vector normal to the curve at abscissa s. Minimization of (2) with steepest gradient descent method is desired in order to solve (3). For this, one assumes the curve depends on time t and is denoted as $v(s, t)$. The following equation is iteratively solved:

$$\frac{\partial v(s, t)}{\partial t \vec{N}} = \alpha \kappa(s, t) + \beta \frac{\partial^4 v(s, t)}{\partial s^4} - \gamma \nabla \left[|\nabla I(v(s, t))|^2 \right] \tag{4}$$

Starting with the initial shape $v(s, 0)$ at time $t = 0$, one lets the dynamical system evolve until it stabilizes, i.e., $\frac{\partial v(s,t)}{\partial t} = 0$.

In this manner, a LV MR slice gets segmented. Following this approach, segmentation on a few more (four to five) pre-selected slices of a subject is performed. Next, we generate segmentation on the rest of the slices of a subject by following a modified level set procedure in order to build the 3D LV.

3 Generation of Missing Contours

Suppose the initial image u_0 consists of only two concentric regions (u_0^i, u_0^o) of piecewise constant intensity (virtually representation of two contours). The variable curve C located at the boundary of u_0^i should move towards its interior normal and stop on the boundary of the outer contour of u_0^o by minimizing the following energy term [7]

$$F(c_1, c_2, \phi) = -\mu \int_\Omega \delta(\phi(x, y)) |\nabla \phi(x, y)| \, dxdy$$

$$- \lambda_1 \int_\Omega |u_0(x, y) - c_1|^2 H(\phi(x, y)) \, dxdy$$

$$- \lambda_2 \int_\Omega |u_0(x,y) - c_2|^2 (1 - H(\phi(x,y))) \, dx dy$$

where constants c_1, c_2 are the averages of u_0 inside and outside C respectively; $\mu \geq 0$ and $\lambda_1 = \lambda_2 = 1$. For level set formulation of the model, $C \subset \Omega$, C is replaced by ϕ and Heaviside function (H) and Dirac measure δ_0 are used. Euler-Lagrange equation for ϕ is deduced, keeping c_1 and c_2 fixed, and minimizing F with respect to ϕ. Parameterizing the ascent direction by a time t, the equation in $\phi(t, x, y)$ (with $\phi(0, x, y) = \phi_0(x, y)$ defining the initial contour) is

$$\frac{\partial \phi}{\partial t} = \partial_\varepsilon(\phi) \left[-\mu \, div \left(\frac{\nabla \phi}{|\nabla \phi|} \right) + \lambda_1 (u_0 - c_1)^2 + \lambda_2 (u_0 - c_2)^2 \right] = 0 \ in \ (0, \infty) \times \Omega,$$

$$\frac{\partial_\varepsilon(\phi)}{|\nabla \phi|} \frac{\partial \phi}{\partial \vec{n}} = 0 \ on \ \partial \Omega$$

where $\frac{\partial \phi}{\partial \vec{n}}$, $\vec{n}$ denote the normal derivative of ϕ at the boundary and the exterior normal to the boundary $\partial \Omega$ respectively. In this way, the intermediate/missing ones between two contours are extracted keeping the track of ϕ at each iteration while C reaches the boundary of u_0^o.

3.1 Method Summary

A subject, on an average, contains 20 MR slices. First, 4–5 slices (if 5, $S_i, i = 1, \ldots, 5$) of a subject are first empirically selected. These slices are segmented using the proposed method considering the 2nd (smallest) eigenvector of the Laplacian matrix as the optimal cut. Initially, the slice or image is treated as a graph; seed points on both FG and BG determine the probability map. The label map is built by considering the maximum of two probabilities at a node. Finally, gradient operation on the label map determines the coordinates that carry nonzero value as the desired contour coordinates. Next, we generate segmentation on the rest of the slices of the subject by following a level set procedure to build the 3D LV where we keep the record of track changes of a contour (of a slice) until it reaches the next selected slice contour. These recorded tracks are the intermediate contours between the two segmented slices (S_i and S_{i-1}).

4 Results

The proposed segmentation algorithm is implemented on two publicly available databases from two different sources viz., a hospital [3] and MICCAI Grand Challenge 2009 [24], so that a researcher may find it pretty useful for comparison. The ground

Table 1 The employed metrics for quantitative evaluation

Measure	Definition
Hausdorff distance (HD)	Minimum distance between two sets of points
False positive ratio (FPR)	Fragment of pixels incorrectly segmented
False negative ratio (FNR)	Fragment of pixels incorrectly rejected
Mean error rate (MER)	(False positive + false negative)/total samples $\times$ 100
Intra-region (I_h) uniformity	Index of homogeneity inside a region
Specificity (Spec)	True negative/(true negative + false positive)
Precision (Prec)	True positive/(True positive + false positive)
Accuracy (Acc)	(True positive + true negative)/total samples
Sensitivity (Sens)	True positive/(true positive/false negative)
Dice coefficient (DC)	Quantity of overlapping of two contours
Pratt's figure of merit (FOM)	Segmentation accuracy

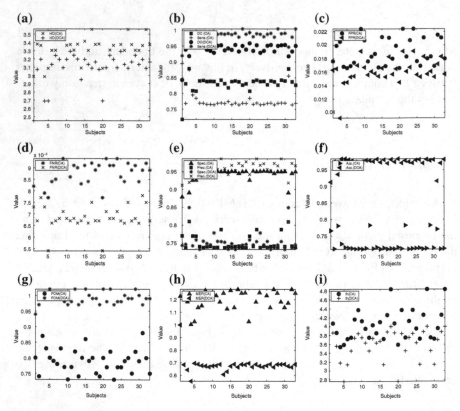

Fig. 1 Values of **a** HD. **b** DC and Sensitivity. **c** FPR. **d** FNR. **e** Specificity and Precision. **f** Accuracy. **g** FOM. **h** MER. **i** I_h

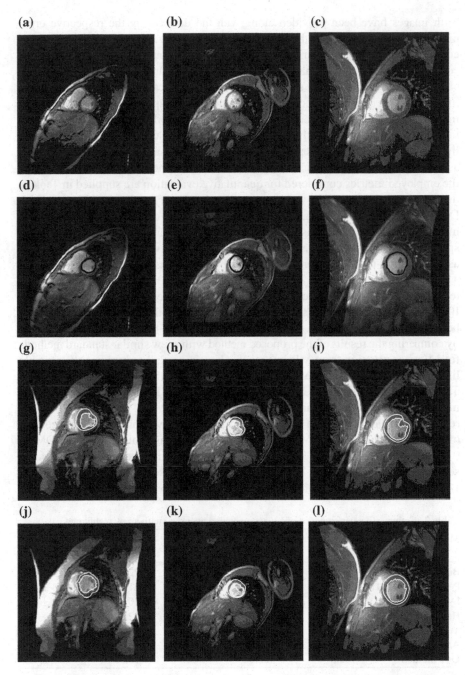

Fig. 2 **a–c** Original images. **d–f** Ground truth images. **g–i** Segmented images due to CA. **j–l** Segmented images due to DCA

truth images have been provided along with the datasets by the respective orga-
nizations. While evaluating the performance, we first examine the performance of
conventional CA which is ruminated in Fig. 2g–i; it may be observed that the resulted
contours rarely match with that of ground truth images. On the other hand, the implication of DCA over the same set of data reflects a significant improvement as shown
in Fig. 2j–l if its qualitative accuracy is examined and compared with the ground truth
images. Simultaneously, it may also be observed that papillary muscles get well segmented by the proposed method which were not possible by traditional CA. Since
the qualitative assessment depends partially on the human judgement, quantitative
assessment becomes a substantiation complement in the performance analysis. Here,
the employed metrics considered for quantitative evaluation are supplied in Table 1;
the measures also include overlap error (Overlap Error), volume difference (Vol.
Diff.), average distance (Avg. Dist.), root mean square distance (RMS Dist.), and
maximum distance (Max. Dist.); as per the definitions of these measures, the corresponding values of these measures along with the first five of the Table 1 should be
as minimum as possible where as that of rest should be as maximum as possible for
a good segmentation output. The quantitative results of 3D image segmentation are
tested on 33 subjects each from both the datasets and the average is given in Fig. 1.
If each figure is carefully observed, the proposed method seems to have performed
better over conventional CA. Subsequently, we evaluate the segmentation accuracy
by comparing the results of the proposed method with a few similar standard methods
for LV reconstruction from MR images that have reportedly overcome the possible
limitations of state of the art MR image segmentation methods; this is summarized in
Table 2. Furthermore, on MICCAI dataset [24], the mean Dice metric (DM in %) and
mean of mean absolute distance (MAD) are found to be 92.4 ± 1.3 and 1.6 ± 0.7,
respectively (values indicate the mean and standard deviation). As reference, one
of the best methods [4] of MICCAI 2009 challenge has achieved a mean DM of
91 ± 0.4 and mean MAD of 2.96 ± 1.09. The average time required to perform the
segmentation is 6 s by a 2GB RAM and core2duo processor on a single CMR image.

Table 2 Comparative performance of LV segmentation accuracy with a few techniques

Method	Overlap error	Vol. Diff. (mm)	Avg. Dist. (mm)	Max. Dist. (mm)	Dice metric (%)
Ben et al. [5]	9.52	0.58	1.46	22.32	86.4 ± 0.8
Pednekar et al. [31]	8.75	0.56	1.39	21.43	88.3 ± 0.6
Lynch et al. [22]	7.87	0.55	1.34	20.67	89.0 ± 0.7
Hae et al. [13]	9.91	0.61	1.49	22.89	85.7 ± 1.1
Yun et al. [42]	7.21	0.45	1.29	20.12	89.4 ± 0.9
Abouzar et al. [1]	7.06	0.43	1.23	19.41	90.4 ± 1.1
Our method	**6.83**	**0.31**	**1.03**	**16.96**	92.3 ± 1.2

5 Conclusions and Future Work

Simple and efficient segmentation methods are always desirable to the radiologists that provide clear shape description of the left ventricle. There are many automated 3D segmentation techniques to the date; but these may turn futile if a clinician desires to move to a specific slice based on the segmentation output or interest. This paper has presented a semi-automatic segmentation algorithm for volumetric LV reconstruction from a few MR slices. The major strength of this work is the integration of snakes into the cellular automaton approach which provides a certain control over the boundary smoothness and potentially prevents smaller leakages. The evaluation also shows a clear benefit to some other similar image segmentation methods. In future, we plan to incorporate this method with various body organs in different modalities.

References

1. Abouzar E, Athanasios K, Amin K, Nassir N (2013) Segmentation by retrieval with guided random walks: application to left ventricle segmentation in MRI. Med Image Anal 17:236–253
2. Adalsteinsson D, Sethian J (1995) A fast level set method for propagating interfaces. J Comput Phys 118:269–277
3. Andre A, Tsotsos J (2008) Efficient and generalizable statistical models of shape and appearance for analysis of CMRI. Med Image Anal 12:335–357
4. Ayed I, Punithakumar K, Li S, Islam A (2009) Left ventricle segmentation via graph cut distribution. In: MICCAI Grand Challenge, Springer, pp 901–909
5. Ben Ayed I, Li S, Ross I (2009) Embedding overlap priors in variational left ventricle tracking. IEEE Trans Med Imaging 28:1902–1913
6. Boykov Y, Jolly MP (2001) Interactive graph cuts for optimal boundary and region segmentation of objects in n-d images. In: ICCV, vol 1, pp 105–112
7. Chan T, Vese L (2001) Active contours without edges. IEEE Trans Image Process 10(2):266–277
8. Dakua S (2011) Performance divergence with data discrepancy: a review. Artif Intell Rev 1:1–27
9. Domany E, Kinzel W (1984) Equivalence of cellular automata to ising models and directed percolation. Phys Rev Lett 53:311–314
10. Frangi A, Niessen W, Viergever M (2001) Three dimensional modeling for functional analysis of cardiac images: a review. IEEE Trans Med Imaging 20(1):2–25
11. Gomes J, Faugeras O (2000) Reconciling distance functions and level sets. J Vis Commun Image Represent 11:209–223
12. Grady L (2006) Random walks for image segmentation. IEEE Trans Pattern Anal Mach Intell 28(11):1–17
13. Hae-Yeoun L, Codella N, Cham M, Weinsaft J, Wang Y (2010) Automatic left ventricle segmentation using iterative thresholding and an active contour model with adaptation on short-axis cardiac MRI. TBME 57:905–913
14. Heimann T et al (2009) Comparison and evaluation of methods for LV segmentation from MR datasets. IEEE Trans Med Imaging 28:1251–1265
15. Herman G, Odhner D (1991) Performance evaluation of an iterative image reconstruction algorithm for positron emission tomography. IEEE Trans Med Imaging 10(3):336–346
16. Ilya P, Alan S, Hamid K (2000) Image segmentation and edge enhancement with stabilized inverse diffusion equations. IEEE Trans Image Process 9(2):256–266

17. Jianbo S, Malik J (2000) Normalized cuts and image segmentation. IEEE Trans Pattern Anal Mach Intell 22(8):888–905
18. Kass M, Witkin A, Terzopolous D (1988) Snakes: active contour models. Int J Comput Vision 4:321–331
19. Krzysztof C, Jayaram U, Falcao A, Miranda P (2012) Fuzzy connectedness image segmentation in graph cut formulation: a linear-time algorithm and a comparative analysis. Math Imaging Vis 44:375–398
20. Li C, Xu C, Gui C, Fox M (2005) Level set formulation without re-initialization: a new variational formulation. Proc IEEE CVPR 1:430–436
21. Lorenzo M, Sanchez G, Mohiaddin R, Rueckert D (2002) Atlas-based segmentation and tracking of 3D cardiac MR images using non-rigid registration. In: MICCAI 2002. LNCS, vol 2488. Springer, Heidelberg, pp 642–650
22. Lynch M, Ghita O, Whelan PF (2008) Segmentation of the left ventricle of the heart in 3-D+t MRI data using an optimized nonrigid temporal model. IEEE Trans Med Imaging 27:195–203
23. Malladi R, Sethian J, Vemuri B (1995) Shape modeling with front propagation: a level set approach. IEEE Trans Pattern Anal Mach Intell 17:158–175
24. MICCAI (2009) Grand Challenge. www.smial.sri.utoronto.ca/LV_Challenge
25. Michael L, Ovidiu G, Paul W (2008) Segmentation of the left ventricle of the heart in 3-D+t MRI data. IEEE Trans Med Imaging 27(2):195–203
26. Mortensen EN, Barrett WA (1998) Interactive segmentation with intelligent scissors. Graphical Models Image Process 60:349–384
27. Nuzillard D, Lazar C (2007) Partitional clustering techniques for multi-spectral image segmentation. J Comput 2(10):1–8
28. Osher S, Sethian J (1988) Fronts propagating with curvature dependent speed: algorithms based on Hamilton-Jacobi formulation. J Comput Phys 79:12–49
29. Paragios N (2003) A level set approach for shape-driven segmentation and tracking of the left ventricle. IEEE Trans Med Imaging 22(6):773–776
30. Pednekar K, Muthupillai R, Flamm S, Kakadiaris I (2006) Automated left ventricular segmentation in cardiac MRI. IEEE Trans Biomed Eng 53(7):1425–1428
31. Pednekar A, Kurkure U, Muthupillai R, Flamm S, Kakadiaris I (2006) Automated LV segmentation in CMRI. TBME 53:1425–1428
32. Pluempitiwiriyawej C, Moura J, Wu Y, Ho C (2005) STACS: new active contour scheme for cardiac MR image segmentation. IEEE Trans Med Imaging 24(5):593–603
33. Rezaee M, Zwet P, Lelieveldt B, Geest R, Reiber J (2000) A multiresolution image segmentation technique based on pyramidal segmentation and fuzzy Clustering. IEEE Trans Image Process 9(7):1238–1248
34. Rother C, Kolmogorov V, Blake A (2004) Grabcut – interactive foreground extraction using iterated graph cuts. In: ACM SIGGRAPH, 2004
35. Song W, Jeffrey S (2003) Segmentation with ratio cut. IEEE Trans Pattern Anal Mach Intell 25(6):675–694
36. Sum K, Paul C (2008) Vessel extraction under non-uniform illumination: a level set approach. IEEE Trans Biomed Eng 55(1):358–360
37. Surendra R (1995) Contour extraction from CMRI studies using snakes. IEEE Trans Med Imaging 14(2):328–338
38. Tood M (1996) The expectation maximization algorithm. IEEE Signal Process Mag 13(6): 47–60
39. Vanzella W, Torre V (2006) A versatile segmentation procedure. IEEE Trans Syst Man Cybern Part C 36(2):366–378
40. Vezhnevets V, Konouchine V (2005) Growcut – interactive multi-label n-d image segmentation by cellular automata. In: Proceedings of Graphicon 2005, pp 150–156
41. Warfield S, Dengler J, Zaers J, Guttmann C, Gil W, Ettinger J, Hiller J, Kikinis R (1995) Automatic identification of grey matter structures from MRI to improve the segmentation of white matter lesions. J Imag Guided Surg 1:326–338
42. Yun Z, Papademetris X, Sinusas A, Duncan J (2010) Segmentation of the left ventricle from cardiac MR images using a subject-specific dynamical model. IEEE Trans Med Imaging 29:669–687

Minimally Interactive MRI Segmentation for Subject-Specific Modelling of the Tongue

Negar M. Harandi, Rafeef Abugharbieh and Sidney Fels

Abstract Subject-Specific biomechanical modelling of the human tongue is beneficial for investigating the inter-subject variability in the physiology of the speech, chewing and swallowing. Delineation of the tongue tissue from MRI is essential for modelling, but still remains a challenge due to the lack of definitive boundary features. In this paper, we propose a minimally interactive inter-subject mesh-to-image registration scheme to tackle 3D segmentation of the tongue from MR volumes. An exemplar expert-delineated template is deformed to match the target volume, constrained based on a shape matching regularization technique. We enable effective minimal user interaction by incorporating additional boundary labels in areas where automatic segmentation is deemed inadequate. We validate our method on 12 normal-subjects. Results indicate an average dice overlap of 0.904 with the ground truth, achieved within 3 min of the expert interaction.

1 Introduction

Speech, chewing and swallowing are critical and complex neuromuscular functions. Various associated disorders result in medical complications that, if not properly treated, may significantly degrade the quality of life of those afflicted. The tongue is the primary organ in the oropharynx and plays an essential role in oropharyngeal functions. It consists of interwoven muscle fibres that undergo a wide range of

N. M. Harandi (✉) · R. Abugharbieh · S. Fels
Department of Electrical and Computer Engineering, University of British Columbia,
Vancouver, Canada
e-mail: negarm@ece.ubc.ca

R. Abugharbieh
e-mail: rafeef@ece.ubc.ca

S. Fels
e-mail: ssfels@ece.ubc.ca

J. M. R. S. Tavares et al. (eds.), *Bio-Imaging and Visualization for Patient-Customized Simulations*, Lecture Notes in Computational Vision and Biomechanics 13,
DOI: 10.1007/978-3-319-03590-1_5, © Springer International Publishing Switzerland 2014

muscular contractions and relaxations whose exact timings and levels of activation are still unknown [1].

Computer-aided modelling of the oropharyngeal structures is beneficial for 3D visualization, and for the understanding of the associated physiology. Generic bio-mechanical models of the Oral, Pharyngeal, and Laryngeal (OPAL) structures are adopted into the ArtiSynth framework [2]. Further expansion of this generic platform, to encompass individualized information, will allow investigation of the subject-specific variability in the morphology and physiology of the region. It will also facilitate future development of the patient-specific platform, in medical settings, which will be aimed at assisting in the diagnosis and treatment planning of speech and swallowing disorders.

Existing biomechanical models of the human tongue [3–5] are generic and do not provide any individualized information. They have been hand-sculpted and simplified to meet the requirements of the simulation platforms. Moreover, their generation workflow is highly manual, tedious, non-trivial and hence, not suitable for creating subject-specific models. Further automation of modelling and simulation procedures is in high demand, and essential for overcoming the associated prohibitive costs [6].

Magnetic Resonance Imaging is a sensitive tool for the analysis of soft tissues in the oropharynx without introducing any known risks. While dynamic, cine and tagged MRI provide insight into the physiology of the tongue, its detailed muscle structure should be inspected through static MRI. High-resolution static MR volumes require a long acquisition time, which leads to involuntary movement of the tongue and, hence, introduces severe motion artifacts. 2D acquisition can provide a refined depiction of the tongue in the acquired plane, but the through-plane resolution is low, and inadequate for most of the volumetric analyses. Super-resolution reconstruction techniques have been introduced to generate isotropic MR volumes from orthogonal slice stacks acquired sequentially [7, 8]. Recently, Woo et al. were able to reconstruct isotropic, high resolution, static MRI volumes of the tongue [9], which provides a great opportunity for intuitive three-dimensional modelling purposes.

Few biomechanical meshing algorithms try to directly generate the subject-specific mesh from image data. The popular voxel-based method [10], identifies the corresponding voxels by thresholding, before transforming them into cubic elements in the final mesh. The method is fully automated, general and robust; however, it lacks the efficient descriptors for identifying the soft-tissues in MRI. In addition, the final mesh suffers from the jagged boundaries and needs to be smoothened, which in turn will cause surface shrinkage and generation of ill-conditioned elements. Other methods rely on organ contours or the surface mesh [11, 12]. Therefore, the modelling process in 3D consists of two consecutive phases of segmentation, and volume mesh generation. The overall efficiency of the process is highly dependant on the accuracy and degree of automation in each phase.

Accurate delineation of the tongue from MRI remains a challenge, due to the lack of definitive boundary features separating many of the adjacent soft-tissues. Manual segmentation produces accurate results, but is prohibitively time-consuming and tedious. General-purpose interactive tools can ease the task, however, they still require significant amounts of user interaction. Previous reported works on segmentation of the oropharyngeal structures focus on 2D MRI slices [13–15]. However, 3D reconstruction of the tongue shape from its sparse 2D segmented contours is not straight-forward. Also, these methods ignore delineation of the tongue at its base and its contact with the epiglottis, hyoid bone and salivary glands, where segmentation is a challenge due fusion into the neighbouring tissues (see Fig. 3 for more details).

Quite recently, Lee et al. proposed a semi-automatic workflow for 3D segmentation of the tongue in dynamic MRI [16]. Their dataset consists of three orthogonal stacks of 2D MR slices, captured in 26 time frames for two English speaking subjects. Their proposed method requires user-given seeds in few slice images (in space) and frames (in time). It then automatically propagates the seeds to the other frames and slices using a deformable image-to-image registration technique, previously proposed by Woo et al. [9]. The seeds are further fed to Random Walker [17] as the core segmentation algorithm. The average overlap of dice = 0.9 was reported with manual segmentation, measured over all 52 volumes (26 time frame × 2 subjects).

Although the aforementioned method proposed by Lee et al. [16], is very useful for motion analysis of the tongue, the different nature of cine and static MRI makes the method inefficient for accurate segmentation of a single high resolution static MRI volume. Figure 1 compares the two datasets. As it can be noticed, the tongue displays a uniform texture in cine-MRI, which justifies the use of Random Walker algorithm. However, this is not the case for static MRI where salivary glands, muscle

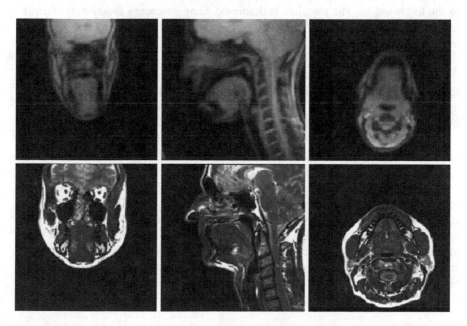

Fig. 1 Quality of the image in Cine-MRI [16] (*top*) versus high resolution static MRI [9] (*bottom*). From *left* to *right* mid-coronal, mid-sagittal and mid-axail slices. Both dataset were acquired in similar orthogonal stacks and reconstructed using the same method [9]

and fat tissue are distinguishable from one another, in high resolution. We believe such detailed anatomical information is essential for biomechanical modelling of the tongue, and, hence, further automation of the segmentation process should be addressed to facilitate the subject-specific workflow. Therefore, in this chapter, we propose a minimally interactive mesh-to-image registration framework to tackle full 3D segmentation of the tongue from static high resolution MR volumes.

2 Related Work

Efficient incorporation of the prior knowledge facilitates the soft-tissue segmentation. Shape constraints have been embedded into level-set framework [18–20], further equipped with trained distance maps [21]. In addition, statistical methods such as the *active shape models* [22], have been widely explored to encompass intra- and inter-subject morphological discrepancies. However, the cardinality of the training set is proportional to the degree of natural variability of the organ shape. For example, Heimann et al. selected 32 subjects out of 86 to train their 3D reference model of 2562 equally distributed landmarks, used for segmentation of the liver in CT volumes [23]. Unfortunately, such a large dataset is currently not available for tongue MRI volumes.

As an alternative, the prior knowledge may be formulated in a template, registered to the target image. The template is deformed using an energy functional, optimizing for the likelihood of the image-features, such as intensity inside the region of interest and its background. Saddi et al. used a template matching procedure as the complementary step to their liver segmentation process, in order to compensate for the limitations of their learning set [24]. Somphone et al. transformed their binary template, subject to conformity constraints between local patches [25]. In a different approach, Gilles et al. used explicit shape representation of the template to segment the musculoskeletal structures out of MR images [26]. The mesh deformation was regularized based on an expanded version of a computer animation technique called *shape matching* [27]. The method was shown to efficiently approximate large soft-tissue elastic deformations.

Despite successful use of the shape prior, automatic segmentation is still challenging in low-contrast medical images of the soft-tissue. The effective and minimal interactivity schemes will provide higher reliability for clinical applications, while keeping the cost of interaction reasonable. Freedman et al. combined shape prior and interactivity in a graph cut framework in 2D [28]. Recently, Somphone et al. incorporated user input as inside/outside labelled points to improved the robustness and accuracy of a non-rigid implicit template deformation [29].

3 Proposed Methods

The overall pipeline of the proposed method is shown in Fig. 2. The source model is delineated by a dental expert from the source image and then deformed to match the target volume (loop 1). We further deploy an effective, minimal user interaction mechanism to help attain higher clinical acceptance (loop 2). Both loops in Fig. 2 have access to and are able to update the current position of the surface nodes, stored in the module called mechanical state, simultaneously. This provides real-time interaction with the surface evolution. The method was fully implemented under the Simulation Open Framework Architecture (SOFA) [30], an open-source modular framework based on C++. This allows for the registration algorithm to be interpreted as a real-time simulation process during which the source model iteratively deforms to match the target configuration starting from its initial position.

3.1 Mesh-to-Volume Registration

Mesh-to-Volume registration, as described in loop 1 of Fig. 2, consists of two modules: intensity profile-based registration and shape matching regularization. We use a Pair-and-Smooth approach [31] to minimize propagation of noise to the final result. Hence, the mesh is deformed in two steps; first, the image forces move the vector of reference vertex positions, x^r, to the vector of current positions, $x(t)$; second, the deformation is smoothened by applying the relevant internal forces, $f^i(t) = \tilde{x} - x(t)$, where $\tilde{x}$ is the new regularized goal positions.

Intensity Profile Registration: We use image-based external forces to steer the mesh toward the target boundaries. For each node at position x on the surface, the external force at time t is calculated by $f^e(t) = \alpha_e(x' - x(t))$ where α_e is the stiffness and x' denotes the new location of the node. The search for x' is performed within a

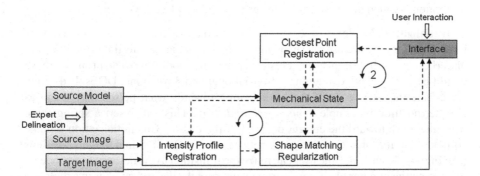

Fig. 2 Proposed pipeline: Iterative loop (1) includes the mesh-to-image registration modules. Iterative loop (2) incorporates potential user-interactive boundary labelling

pre-defined range of inward and outward steps at the direction normal to the surface. At each iteration, x' is selected to be the point which maximizes a local similarity measure between the source and target image volumes. Our algorithm matches the gradient intensity patches of pre-defined length. Normalized cross correlation was used as the similarity metric.

Shape Matching Regularization: To regularize the mesh deformation, we apply the extended version of the shape matching algorithm previously introduced in the context of musculoskeletal structures by Gilles et al. [26]. The underlying mesh is subdivided into clusters of nodes, ζ_i, defined around each node i on the surface as $\zeta_i = \{j : d(x_i, x_j) < s\}$, where d is the Euclidean distance and s is the predefined cluster size (or radius). Then, for each cluster ζ_i, the algorithm approximates the local deformation of the nodes with a rigid transform $\mathbf{T}_i$, between $x(t)$ and the reference position x^r, as in $\tilde{x} = \mathbf{T}x^r$. The least square estimation of $\mathbf{T}_i$ is obtained by minimizing the following metric: $\sum_{j \in \zeta_i} m_j \parallel \mathbf{T}x_j^r - x_j \parallel$ where m_j represents the mass weight of each particle in the cluster. This in turn will update the goal position of each node in the cluster.

Due to the overlapping nature of the clusters, each vertex may obtain different goal positions from the different clusters it may belong to, which we subsequently combine into an average position. The final goal position is used to calculate the corresponding internal forces which are then averaged and applied to all the vertices of each cluster. Here, shape matching acts as an elastic force that is proportional to the strain whereas updating the reference positions at each time step will simulate plastic deformations. To summarize, one iteration of the registration technique using shape matching involves the following steps:

1. Calculate external forces f^e.
2. Calculate shape matching forces f^i:

    a. For each cluster ζ_i, compute $\mathbf{T}_i = argmin \sum_{j \in \zeta_i} m_j \parallel \mathbf{T}x_j^r - x_j - f_j^e \parallel^2$

    b. Average goal positions $\tilde{x}_i = \sum_i (\mathbf{T})x_i^r / |\zeta_i|$ for each vertex i.

3. Evolve node positions: $x = \tilde{x}$.
4. Optionally, update reference positions to simulate plasticity: $x_r = x$.

Initialization Mode: In order to drag the mesh close to the position of the tongue in the target image, we use the shape matching technique but this time we model the underlxying mesh with just one cluster. Hence, the bodily movement of the mesh would be purely rigid, containing 3 translational and 3 rotational DOFs. If desired, we enable the user to guide the initialization towards what he/she may deem as a better position by simple *mouse-click and drag*. This will insert a spring force from the mesh toward the current position of the cursor. This initialization scheme compensates for large displacements between the initial and final tongue positions (see Fig. 4). At any time, the user can make the transition to the deformation mode by increasing the number of clusters, through entering the desired number in a dialogue box and pressing a button.

3.2 User Interaction

We incorporate an effective minimal user interaction mechanism to guarantee a satisfactory result to the end user (see loop 2 in Fig. 2). At any time during the registration process, the user is free to inspect the orthogonal cut-planes of the deforming mesh, overlaid on the corresponding 2D sections of the target image. The user may provide additional boundary labels by simple clicking in any area where automatic segmentation is deemed inadequate. As soon as a new boundary voxel is clicked, the algorithm searches for the closest surface node on the mesh and inserts a spring force between these two points. The closest points on the surface will get updated in each iteration of the mesh deformation. We empirically used a predefined stiffness of about 10^4 in all implementations. Stiffness values of higher order of magnitude may cause instability and hence are avoided.

4 Results and Discussion

The proposed method was validated on 12 normal subjects (5 females–7 males) with their tongue at supine rest position. For each subject, an isotropic volume was reconstructed from three sagittal, coronal, and axial stacks of MRI slices. The MRI scanner was a Siemens 3.0T, Tim Treo system with an 8-channel head and neck coil. The size of each MRI stack was $256 \times 256 \times z$ (z ranges from 10 to 24) with 0.94 mm $\times$ 0.94 mm in-plane resolution and 3mm slice thickness. Isotropic resolution of 0.94 mm was achieved after volume reconstruction. Details of data acquisition and reconstruction technique can be found in [9].

All 12 subjects were manually segmented under the supervision of our dental expert collaborator using the interactive tool TurtleSeg [32] (see Fig. 3). The results were used both as the source surface mesh in the proposed segmentation method and as the ground truth for validation purposes. The segmented surface for each volume included all the internal muscles of tongue as well as the digastric, geniohyoid and hyoglossus muscles. It excluded the hyoid and mandible bone, epiglottis and salivary glands. We cut the mylohyoid, palatoglossus and styloglossus muscles following the contour of the tongue. In addition, the tongue tissue above the line between the epiglottis and hyoid bone was included. The manual segmentation took about 3–5 h for each subject.

Due to the large difference between the general shapes of the tongues in male and female subjects, we categorized the subjects into two groups of *female* and *male* anatomy. For each volume in each group, the segmentation was repeated by iterating the source on other members of the corresponding group. In each case, the dental expert was asked to interact with the segmentation for the minimum of 1 and maximum of 3 min. It should be noted that registration between two groups is also possible but requires more intervention of the user. The volume overlap was calculated before and after the interaction. We used the dice coefficient as a measure

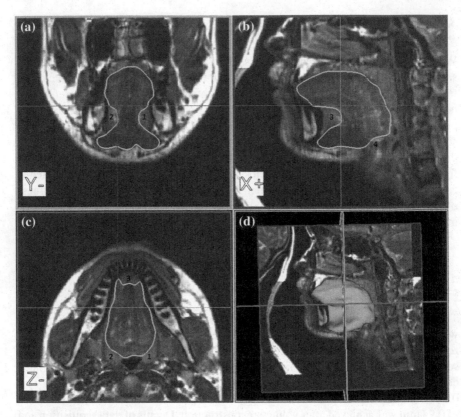

Fig. 3 Ground truth segmented by dental expert in TurtlesSeg [32]. **a** Mid-coronal, **b** Mid-sagittal and **c** Mid-axial slices shown with **d** 3D volume of the tongue. Salivary glands (*labels 1–3*) and hyoid bone (*label 4*) had been excluded

of volume overlap between the result (A) and the ground truth (B), reported as a percentage:

$$Dice = 2\frac{|A \cap B|}{|A| + |B|} \times 100.$$

Table 1-top shows the results before and after user interaction for group 1, which included six normal male volunteers. We noticed that anatomy of one male subject matched better with the female group, therefore, it was excluded from group 1 and added to group 2. The average dice, measured on all the volumes in the group, improved from 88.93 ± 1.38 to 90.42 ± 0.39 after expert interaction. The mean of the inter-subject standard deviation (STD) also dropped from 1.87 ± 0.60 to 0.60 ± 0.16. Table 1-bottom shows the volume overlap for group 2 (females). The average metric in the group is 87.68 ± 1.66, before, and 90.44 ± 0.40, after interaction. The mean of the measured STD also changes from 1.5 ± 0.35 to 0.63 ± 0.24. Figure 4 shows the evolution of the mesh for one male subject, through different stages of

Table 1 Average dice coefficients before (white) and after (grey) expert interaction time of 2 ± 1 min: Results for the male group (top) and female group (bottom)

Data #	1	2	3	4	5	6
Mean	87.73	86.06	89.44	89.50	88.02	86.85
STD	1.73	2.06	0.84	1.83	2.06	2.69
Mean	90.32	89.87	90.93	90.80	90.26	90.34
STD	0.57	0.47	0.40	0.86	0.63	0.64
Data #	1	2	3	4	5	6
Mean	86.96	87.87	88.63	89.71	88.08	84.83
STD	1.16	1.40	1.89	1.10	1.91	1.54
Mean	90.00	90.35	90.64	90.90	90.80	89.96
STD	0.26	0.66	0.75	0.98	0.62	0.50

the proposed algorithm. First, the source mesh is directly uploaded into the target space (1st row). Second, the difference in position of the tongue, between the source and the target space, is compensated during the initialization step (2nd row). Next, the user enables the registration by increasing the number of clusters (3rd row). The circled regions denote the areas that the registration was deemed to be inaccurate. Further, the user clicks on the correct boundaries in real-time to modify the mesh (4th row).

The manual segmentation used as the ground truth is likely to be fuzzy and uncertain in problematic regions, e.g. at the boundary of the hyoid bone and the salivary glands. However, modelling requisites prohibit the segmentation to include bones and non-muscle soft tissues. To assess such uncertainty, we designed an experiment in which the same dental expert was asked to repeat the same manual segmentation after 10 days, while avoiding referring to the first set. The result showed a volume overlap of dice = 91 between the two manually segmented volumes. We argue that this uncertainty imposes an upper limit of about the same value on the achievable automated segmentation volume overlap. In fact, while expert interaction resulted in about 7 improvement for dice values of as low as 83, the improvement was less than 1 for values as high as 90.

Implementation Details: All the parameters were fixed in all experiments. We unified the number of surface nodes to 2502. For the intensity profile registration module, the length of the profiles was set to 50 pixels, centred on the investigated voxel. The search range was 5 voxels, inward and outward, in the normal direction to the mesh surface. The stiffness coefficient, α_e, was set to 1. For shape matching regularization, the results without user interaction were similar with the number of clusters ranging between 200 and 500. We set this variable to 300. To attain high flexibility, the radius of all clusters were set to 1.

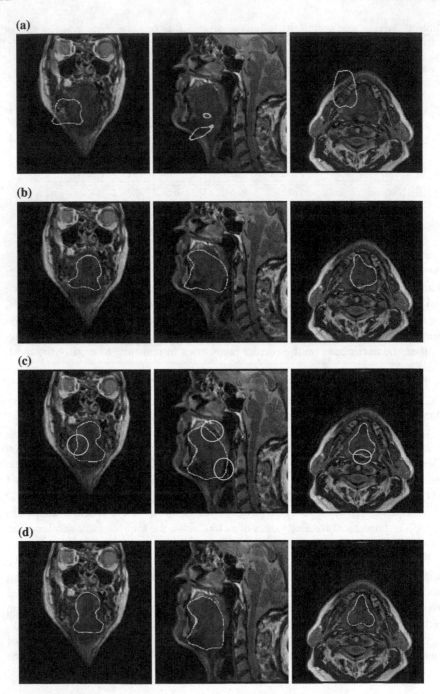

Fig. 4 Mesh evolution during the segmentation process in mid-coronal (*left*), mid-sagittal (*middle*) and mid-axial (*right*) slices. Position of the tongue in the initial configuration (**a**), after initialization phase (**b**), after mesh-to-volume registration (**c**) and after user interaction (**d**). The *red circles* in (**c**) denote the areas in which user input is deemed necessary

5 Conclusions and Future Work

In this chapter, we tackled the challenging problem of automated 3D segmentation of the tongue from isotropic MRI volumes. Previous works included delineation of the tongue contours at its surface in 2D MRI slices. We adapted an inter-subject registration framework using a shape matching-based regularization technique. The method was combined with an instant force-based user interaction mechanism which attracts the model towards user-provided boundary labels. We were able to achieve average segmentation accuracy of dice = 0.904 ± 0.004, within few minutes of expert interaction. Also, the total running time is about 5 min comparing to about 5 h of manual segmentation. Our future work will integrate the proposed segmentation method within a subject-specific FE modelling framework, aimed for speech and swallowing studies.

Acknowledgments This work was supported in part by NSERC, CHRP and NCE GRAND. The authors would like to thank the collaborators from *Dental School* at *University of Maryland*— Professor *Maureen Stone* and Dr. *Jonghye Woo*—for providing the MRI dataset. Also, our dental expert Dr. *Ho Beom Kwon* is greatly acknowledged for supervising the validation process.

References

1. Steele CM, Van Lieshout P (2009) Tongue movements during water swallowing in healthy young and older adults. J Speech Lang Hear Res 52(5):1255
2. Lloyd JE, Stavness I, Fels S (2012) ARTISYNTH: a fast interactive biomechanical modeling toolkit combining multibody and finite element simulation. Soft tissue biomechanical modeling for computer assisted surgery. Springer, Berlin, Heidelberg
3. Badin P, Bailly G, Reveret L, Baciu M, Segebarth C, Savariaux C (2002) Three-dimensional linear articulatory modeling of tongue, lips and face, based on MRI and video images. J Phonetics 30(3):533–553
4. Gerard JM, Wilhelms-Tricarico R, Perrier P, Payan Y (2006) A 3D dynamical biomechanical tongue model to study speech motor control. arXiv preprint physics/0606148
5. Sonomura M, Mizunuma H, Numamori T, Michiwaki H, Nishinari K (2011) Numerical simulation of the swallowing of liquid bolus. J Texture Stud 42(3):203–211
6. Neal ML, Kerckhoffs R (2010) Current progress in patient-specific modelling. Briefings Bioinform 11(1):111–126
7. Peled S, Yehezkel Y (2001) Superresolution in MRI: application to human white matter fiber tract visualization by diffusion tensor imaging. Magn Reson Med 45(1):29–35
8. Bai Y, Xiao H, Prince JL (2004) Super-resolution reconstruction of MR brain images. Proceedings of 38th annual conference on information sciences and systems (CISS?04)
9. Woo J, Murano E, Stone M, Prince J (2012) Reconstruction of high resolution tongue volumes from MRI. IEEE Trans Biomed Eng 6(1):1–25
10. Keyak JH, Meagher JM, Skinner HB, Mote CD (1990) Automated three-dimensional finite element modelling of bone: a new method. J Biomed Eng 12(5):389–397
11. Teo JCM, Chui CK, Wang ZL, Ong SH, Yan CH, Wang SC, Wong HK, Teoh SH (2007) Heterogeneous meshing and biomechanical modeling of human spine. Med Eng Phys 29(2):277–290
12. Bucki M, Nazari MA, Payan Y (2010) Finite element speaker-specific face model generation for the study of speech production. Comput Methods Biomech Biomed Eng 13(4):459–467

13. Bresch E, Narayanan S (2009) Region segmentation in the frequency domain applied to upper airway real-time magnetic resonance images. IEEE Trans Med Imaging 28(3):323–338
14. Peng T, Kerrien E, Berger MO (2010) A shape-based framework to segmentation of tongue contours from MRI data. In: IEEE international conference on acoustics speech and signal processing (ICASSP), IEEE Press, pp 662–665
15. Eryildirim A, Berger MO (2011) A guided approach for automatic segmentation and modeling of the vocal tract in MRI images. In: European signal processing conference (EUSIPCO)
16. Lee J, Woo J, Xing F, Murano EZ, Stone M, Prince JL (2013) Semi-automatic segmentation of the tongue for 3D motion analysis with dynamic MRI. In: IEEE 10th international symposium on biomedical imaging (ISBI), IEEE Press
17. Grady L (2006) Random walks for image segmentation. IEEE Trans Pattern Anal Mach Intell 28(11):1768–1783
18. Leventon M E, Grimson WEL, Faugeras O (2000) Statistical shape influence in geodesic active contours. Computer vision and pattern recognition. In: Proceedings, IEEE conference on 1
19. Tsai A, Yezzi A, Wells W, Tempany C, Tucker D, Fan A, Grimson WE, Willsky A (2003) A shape-based approach to the segmentation of medical imagery using level sets. Med Imaging IEEE Trans 22(2):137–154
20. Foulonneau A, Charbonnier P, Heitz F (2009) Multi-reference shape priors for active contours. Int J Comput Vis 81(1):68–81
21. Bresson X, Vandergheynst P, Thiran J (2006) A variational model for object segmentation using boundary information and shape prior driven by the Mumford-Shah functional. Int J Comput Vis 68(2):145–162
22. Cootes TF et al (1995) Active shape models: their training and application. Comput Vis Image Underst 61(1):38–59
23. Heimann T, Münzing S, Meinzer HP (2007) A shape-guided deformable model with evolutionary algorithm initialization for 3D soft tissue segmentation. In: Karssemeijer N, Lelieveldt B (eds) Inf Process Med Imaging 5484:1–10. Springer
24. Saddi KA, Rousson M, Chefd HC, Cheriet F (2007) Global-to-local shape matching for liver segmentation in CT imaging. MICCAI
25. Somphone O, Mory B, Makram-Ebeid S, Cohen L (2008) Prior-based piecewise-smooth segmentation by template competitive deformation using partitions of unity. In: Computer vision? ECCV 2008. Springer, Berlin Heidelberg, pp 628–641
26. Gilles B, Pai D (2008) Fast musculoskeletal registration based on shape matching. In: Metaxas DN, Axe L (eds) MICCAI 2008, LNCS, vol 5242. Springer, Heidelberg, pp 822–829
27. Muller M, Heidelberger B, Teschner M, Gross M (2005) Meshless deformations based on shape matching. ACM Trans Graphics 24(3):471–478. ACM
28. Freedman D, Zhang T (2005) Interactive graph cut based segmentation with shape priors. Computer vision and pattern recognition (2005). IEEE computer society conference on 1, IEEE
29. Mory B, Somphone O, Prevost R, Ardon (2012) Real-Time 3d image segmentation by user-constrained template deformation. In: MICCAI 2012. Springer, Berlin, Heidelberg, pp 561–568
30. SOFA (2013) Simulation open framework architecture. www.sofa-framework.org
31. Cachier P, Ayache N (2001) Regularization in image non-rigid registration: I. Trade-off between smoothness and intensity similarity. Technical report, INRIA
32. Top A, Hamarneh G, Abugharbieh R (2011) Active learning for interactive 3d image segmentation. In: Peters T, Fichtinger L (eds) MICCAI 2011, LNCS, vol 6893. Springer, Heidelberg, pp 603–610

Real-time and Accurate Endoscope Electromagnetic Tracking via Marker-free Registration Based on Endoscope Tip Center

Xiongbiao Luo and Kensaku Mori

Abstract This paper proposes an improved marker-free registration framework that uses the center of an endoscope tip to establish a spatial alignment between an electromagnetic tracker and pre-operative images (e.g., computed tomography). To obtain such an alignment, currently available marker-free registration methods assume that endoscopes are operated along the centerline of hollow organs (e.g., airway trees). However, such an assumption fails easily during clinical interventions. To tackle such an assumption, we estimate the position of the endoscope tip center in terms of each measurement of an electromagnetic sensor that is attached at the endoscope tip since the center position is usually closer to the organ centerline than the sensor measured position. our experimental results from phantom validation demonstrate that our simple idea of using the position of the endoscope tip center to perform the marker-free registration was very effective, reducing the tracking error significantly from at least 6.3 to 4.0 mm compared to currently available methods.

1 Introduction

Medical endoscopes are broadly used in clinical practice for disease diagnosis and surgery, e.g., bronchoscope or endobronchial ultrasound is employed to conduct surgical tools or needles to biopsy pulmonary lymph nodes for pathological analysis during lung cancer diagnosis and staging. Endoscopes usually provide only two-dimensional (2-D) video images without its tip location information. Hence it is somewhat difficult to locate the endoscope tip around target regions during surgical interventions. Endoscope tracking or navigation is actively discussed to tackle such

X. Luo (✉) · K. Mori
Information and Communications Headquarters, Nagoya Unversity, Nagoya 464-8604, Japan
e-mail: xiongbiao.luo@gmail.com

K. Mori
e-mail: kensaku@is.nagoya-u.ac.jp

J. M. R. S. Tavares et al. (eds.), *Bio-Imaging and Visualization for Patient-Customized Simulations*, Lecture Notes in Computational Vision and Biomechanics 13, DOI: 10.1007/978-3-319-03590-1_6, © Springer International Publishing Switzerland 2014

a difficulty of endoscope location [1–5]. It commonly uses 2-D video images and pre-operative computed tomography (CT) images to construct an augmented reality environment where the current location of the endoscope tip can be directly visualized in the pre-operative CT image space. Therefore, it enables physicians to reach any suspicious tumors in a short time and perform any surgical interventions successfully to sample cancerous tissues exactly as physicians expect.

One of currently available strategies to track or navigate the endoscope is to use an electromagnetic tracking (EMT) system with an EMT sensor is attached to the endoscope tip to estimate its movements. Hence, the spatial alignment between the EMT and CT (EMT-CT) image coordinate systems must be established. Current publications have discussed marker-based and marker-free alignment methods. By choosing among five and seven anatomic markers, Schwarz et al. [6] computed the EMT-CT transformation under a patient movement compensation mechanism and showed the fiducial registration error (FRE) about 5.7 mm. A marker-free method was proposed to maximize the percentage of EMT measurements inside the airway volume to obtain the EMT-CT alignment [7]. Such a method suffers from its initial estimation during optimization. Another marker-free approach on the basis of the centerline information of the organ aims to match the EMT measurements to the centerlines [8]. Such a centerline matching method minimizes the distances among the EMT measurements and the centerlines to determine the EMT-CT transformation. Unfortunately, it assumes that the endoscope is operated along the centerlines, which can be easily violated in clinical applications. Generally, marker-free approaches are promising to establish the EMT-CT alignment for endoscope tracking since they need not choose markers in operating rooms.

This work aims to improve the marker-free registration accuracy to precisely determine the EMT-CT transformation to robustly track or navigate an endoscope during surgical interventions. We seek to resolve the assumption of moving endoscopes along organ centerlines [8]. Our idea is to move the EMT sensor position to the endoscope tip center since we believe that the position of the endoscope tip center is generally closer to the centerlines than the position of EMT sensor measurements. Although our idea is simple, it will be proved to very effectively improve the EMT performance in accordance with our experimental results. The highlight of this work is clarified as follows. We proposed an improved marker-free registration approach on the basis of endoscope tip center information for endoscope tracking and navigation. We introduced three strategies: (1) phantom-based calibration using one EMT sensor, (2) using two sensors, and (3) three sensors, to determine the position of the endoscope tip center. An accurate and real-time endoscope tracking can be obtain by our proposed method.

2 Approaches

Our approach consists of three main steps: (1) preprocessing and initialization, (2) computation of the endoscope tip center, and (3) determination of EMT-CT transformation $_{EMT}^{CT}\mathbf{T}$. The three steps of our method are described as follows.

2.1 Preprocessing and Initialization

Since our method uses bronchial structures, we segment the CT images to get the bronchial centerlines and depict all the bronchi by $\mathscr{B} = \{\mathbf{B}_j = (\mathbf{B}_j', \mathbf{B}_j'')\}_{j=1}^{N}$ (bronchus number N and centerline $\mathbf{B}_j$ with start and end points, $\mathbf{B}_j'$, $\mathbf{B}_j''$).

Before computing $_{EMT}^{CT}\mathbf{T}$ in the optimization, we must initialize it. Using trachea centerline $\mathbf{B}_T$, we can select position $\mathbf{q}_{CT} = \mathbf{B}_T'' - \Delta \cdot (\mathbf{B}_T'' - \mathbf{B}_T') \cdot ||\mathbf{B}_T'' - \mathbf{B}_T'||^{-1}$ (Δ is a constant) in the CT images and register $\mathbf{q}_{CT}$ with EMT sensor position $\mathbf{p}_{EMT}$ and orientation $(\mathbf{s}_{EMT}^x, \mathbf{s}_{EMT}^y, \mathbf{s}_{EMT}^z)$ and determine initial estimate $_{EMT}^{CT}\mathbf{T}_0$, which can minimize the Euclidean distance between a number of EMT sensor measurement points or positions and the trachea centerline.

2.2 Endoscope Tip Center Computation

We introduce three strategies, which corresponds to use one sensor, two sensors, and three sensors respectively, to compute the position of the endoscope tip center in the EMT coordinate system, as shown in Fig. 1. The computation of the center position in different strategies is discussed in the following.

We clarify some notations first. Suppose EMT sensor measurement at time i is $\mathbf{m}_i = (\mathbf{p}_i, \mathbf{s}_i^x, \mathbf{s}_i^y, \mathbf{s}_i^z)$, $\mathbf{p}_i$ is the sensor position, and $\mathbf{s}_i^x$, $\mathbf{s}_i^y$, and $\mathbf{s}_i^z$ indicate the sensor orientation in the three directions of x-, y-, and z-axes.

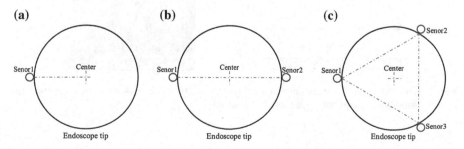

Fig. 1 EMT sensor configurations of using **a** one, **b** two, and **c** three sensors

2.2.1 One Sensor

To compute the center position in case of using one EMT sensor, we require to construct a calibration model, as shown in Fig. 2. We insert the endoscope tip with an EMT sensor into such a model and spin the rotatable cuboid. We collect three measurements of the EMT sensor after rotating about every 120°. We represent these measurements by

$$\mathbf{m}_A = (\mathbf{p}_A, \mathbf{s}_A^x, \mathbf{s}_A^y, \mathbf{s}_A^z), \mathbf{m}_B = (\mathbf{p}_B, \mathbf{s}_B^x, \mathbf{s}_B^y, \mathbf{s}_B^z), \mathbf{m}_C = (\mathbf{p}_C, \mathbf{s}_C^x, \mathbf{s}_C^y, \mathbf{s}_C^z). \quad (1)$$

Based on points $\mathbf{p}_A$, $\mathbf{p}_B$, and $\mathbf{p}_C$, we can determine center $\mathbf{p}_O$ of one circle by solving the following equation:

$$\|\mathbf{p}_O - \mathbf{p}_A\| = \|\mathbf{p}_O - \mathbf{p}_B\| = \|\mathbf{p}_O - \mathbf{p}_C\|, \quad (2)$$

where $\|\cdot\|$ is the Euclidean norm. Since the spatial relationship between the fixed sensor and the endoscope tip center is unchangeable when moving the endoscope, it should satisfy the following condition:

$$\mathbf{p}_A + \Delta_x \mathbf{s}_A^x + \Delta_y \mathbf{s}_A^y + \Delta_z \mathbf{s}_A^z = \mathbf{p}_O. \quad (3)$$

By solving Eq. 3, we can obtain constants Δ_x, Δ_y, and Δ_z which describe the spatial relationship of the sensor and the tip center. Based on Δ_x, Δ_y, and Δ_z, endoscope tip center position $\hat{\mathbf{p}}_i$, which corresponds to measurement $\mathbf{m}_i$ with position $\mathbf{p}_i$ and orientation $(\mathbf{s}_i^x, \mathbf{s}_i^y, \mathbf{s}_i^z)$ at time i, can be determined by:

$$\hat{\mathbf{p}}_i = \mathbf{p}_i + \Delta_x \mathbf{s}_i^x + \Delta_y \mathbf{s}_i^y + \Delta_z \mathbf{s}_i^z. \quad (4)$$

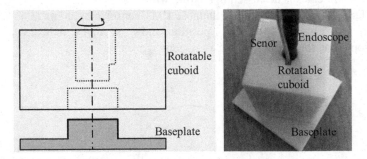

Fig. 2 Our model used for calibrating the relation between the EMT sensor and the endoscope tip center positions in case of only using one EMT sensor

2.2.2 Two Sensors

In case of attaching two sensors at the endoscope tip (Fig. 1b), endoscope tip center position $\hat{\mathbf{p}}_i$ can be easily calculated by:

$$\hat{\mathbf{p}}_i = \frac{\mathbf{p}_i^1 + \mathbf{p}_i^2}{2}, \tag{5}$$

where $\mathbf{p}_i^1$ and $\mathbf{p}_i^2$ are the outputs of two sensors at time i.

2.2.3 Three Sensors

By uniformly attaching three sensors at the endoscope tip, we can solve the following equation to obtain ndoscope tip center position $\hat{\mathbf{p}}_i$:

$$\left\| \hat{\mathbf{p}}_i - \mathbf{p}_i^1 \right\| = \left\| \hat{\mathbf{p}}_i - \mathbf{p}_i^2 \right\| = \left\| \hat{\mathbf{p}}_i - \mathbf{p}_i^3 \right\|, \tag{6}$$

where $\mathbf{p}_i^1$, $\mathbf{p}_i^2$, and $\mathbf{p}_i^3$ are the outputs of three sensors at time i.

2.3 Determination of Transformation $_{EMT}^{CT}\mathbf{T}$

After obtaining endoscope center position $\hat{\mathbf{p}}_i$, we find the closest bronchial centerline $\mathbf{B}_j$ to $\hat{\mathbf{p}}_i$, which is transformed to CT point $_{EMT}^{CT}\mathbf{T} \cdot \hat{\mathbf{p}}_i$ in terms of distance $D(_{EMT}^{CT}\mathbf{T} \cdot \hat{\mathbf{p}}_i, \mathbf{B}_j)$ that is computed by the following equation (Fig. 3):

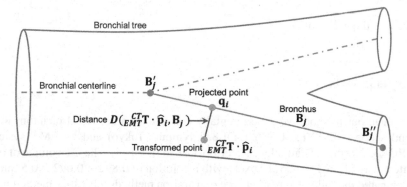

Fig. 3 Assignment of closest centerline $\mathbf{B}_j$ to transformed point $_{EMT}^{CT}\mathbf{T} \cdot \hat{\mathbf{p}}_i$ and obtaining projected point $\mathbf{q}_i$ on basis of distance $\mathbf{L}(_{EMT}^{CT}\mathbf{T} \cdot \hat{\mathbf{p}}_i, \mathbf{B}_j)$

$$D(_{EMT}^{CT}\mathbf{T}\hat{\mathbf{p}}_i, \mathbf{B}_j) = \begin{cases} ||_{EMT}^{CT}\mathbf{T} \cdot \hat{\mathbf{p}}_i - \mathbf{B}_j^{'}|| & \gamma < 0 \\ ||_{EMT}^{CT}\mathbf{T} \cdot \hat{\mathbf{p}}_i - \mathbf{B}_j^{'}|| & \gamma > ||\mathbf{B}_j^{''} - \mathbf{B}_j^{'}|| \ , \\ \sqrt{||_{EMT}^{CT}\mathbf{T} \cdot \hat{\mathbf{p}}_i - \mathbf{B}_j^{'}||^2 - \gamma^2} & otherwise \end{cases} \quad (7)$$

where $\gamma = (_{EMT}^{CT}\mathbf{T} \cdot \hat{\mathbf{p}}_i - \mathbf{B}_j^{'}) \cdot (\mathbf{B}_j^{''} - \mathbf{B}_j^{'}) \cdot ||\mathbf{B}_j^{''} - \mathbf{B}_j^{'}||^{-1}$. After computing the distance between $_{EMT}^{CT}\mathbf{T} \cdot \hat{\mathbf{p}}_i$ and all centerlines $\{\mathbf{B}_j\}_{j=1}^{N}$, we may get several bronchi $\{\mathbf{B}_k, k = 1, 2, 3, \cdots\}$ that have the same closest distance to point $_{EMT}^{CT}\mathbf{T} \cdot \hat{\mathbf{p}}_i$. We further investigate the angle between bronchus direction $(\mathbf{B}_k^{''} - \mathbf{B}_k^{'}) \cdot ||\mathbf{B}_k^{''} - \mathbf{B}_k^{'}||^{-1}$ and sensor running direction $\mathbf{s}_i^z$ to determine optimal centerline $\hat{\mathbf{B}}_i$ by

$$\hat{\mathbf{B}}_i = \arg\min_{\{\mathbf{B}_k\}} \arccos < \frac{\mathbf{B}_k^{''} - \mathbf{B}_k^{'}}{||\mathbf{B}_k^{''} - \mathbf{B}_k^{'}||}, \frac{_{EMT}^{CT}\mathbf{T} \cdot \mathbf{s}_i^z}{||_{EMT}^{CT}\mathbf{T} \cdot \mathbf{s}_i^z||} >, \quad (8)$$

where $<, >$ means the dot product.

After obtaining optimal centerline $\hat{\mathbf{B}}_i$, we project $\hat{\mathbf{p}}_i$ on $\hat{\mathbf{B}}_i$ and calculate projected point $\mathbf{q}_i$ (Fig. 3) by

$$\mathbf{q}_i = \hat{\mathbf{B}}_i^{'} + \frac{(_{EMT}^{CT}\mathbf{T} \cdot \hat{\mathbf{p}}_i - \hat{\mathbf{B}}_i^{'}) \cdot (\hat{\mathbf{B}}_i^{''} - \hat{\mathbf{B}}_i^{'})}{||\hat{\mathbf{B}}_i^{''} - \hat{\mathbf{B}}_i^{'}||} \cdot \frac{(\hat{\mathbf{B}}_i^{''} - \hat{\mathbf{B}}_i^{'})}{||\hat{\mathbf{B}}_i^{''} - \hat{\mathbf{B}}_i^{'}||}. \quad (9)$$

$_{EMT}^{CT}\mathbf{T}$ is eventually determined by minimizing the distance between selected point set $\mathscr{M} = \{\hat{\mathbf{m}}_i = (\hat{\mathbf{p}}_i, \mathbf{s}_i^x, \mathbf{s}_i^y, \mathbf{s}_i^z)\}_{i=1}^{M}$ and projected point set $\mathscr{Q} = \{\mathbf{q}_i\}_{i=1}^{M}$ (EMT sensor output number M):

$$_{EMT}^{CT}\hat{\mathbf{T}} = \arg\min_{\hat{\mathbf{m}}_i \in \mathscr{M}, \mathbf{q}_i \in \mathscr{Q}} \sum_i \frac{||_{EMT}^{CT}\mathbf{T} \cdot \hat{\mathbf{p}}_i - \mathbf{q}_i||}{\hat{r}_i}, \quad (10)$$

where $\hat{r}_i$ is the radius of $\hat{\mathbf{B}}_i$.

3 Experiments

To evaluate our method, we experimentally constructed a bronchial phantom with an endoscope (BF TYPE US260F-OL8, Olympus, Tokyo) and an EMT system (AURORA, Northern Digital Inc, Waterloo, Canada) (Fig. 4). The CT volume of our phantom was $512 \times 512 \times 611$ voxels with resolution of $0.892 \times 0.692 \times 0.5$ mm^3. We compared the following marker-free registration methods: (1) M0, a method proposed by Deguchi et al. [8], (2) M1, using one sensor to calibrate the endoscope tip center (Sect. 2), (3) M2, using two sensors to obtain the tip center (Sect. 2), and (4)

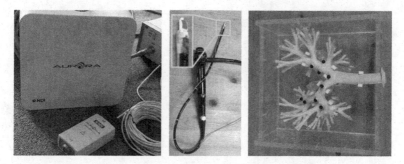

Fig. 4 EMT tracker, endoscope, and phantom used in our experiments

M3, using three sensors to determine the tip sensor center (Sect. 2). We computed the fiducial registration error of $^{CT}_{EMT}\hat{\mathbf{T}}$ using 20 markers on the static phantom:

$$Err = \sum_{e=1}^{E=20} ||^{CT}\mathbf{q}_e - ^{CT}_{EMT}\hat{\mathbf{T}} \cdot \mathbf{p}_e^{EMT}||/E, \tag{11}$$

where we manually determined marker position $^{CT}\mathbf{q}_e$ in the CT images.

4 Results

Table 1 quantifies the fiducial registration error of the four approaches validated by ten experiments. The average registration errors of M0, M1, M2, and M3 were about 6.3, 4.0, 4.3, and 4.7 mm, respectively. Fig. 5 plots the fiducial registration error

Table 1 Quantitative comparison of fiducial registration error from methods of M0, M1, M2, and M3

Experiments	M0 (mm)	M1 (mm)	M2 (mm)	M3
1	6.8	4.1	4.0	4.5
2	7.3	5.1	4.9	5.3
3	5.8	4.2	4.7	5.0
4	7.0	4.1	4.1	4.5
5	4.9	3.4	3.5	4.1
6	6.4	3.7	3.8	4.0
7	7.7	5.0	5.8	6.0
8	5.8	3.5	3.7	4.5
9	6.4	3.9	4.2	5.2
10	5.2	3.9	4.5	4.7
Average	6.3	4.0	4.3	4.7

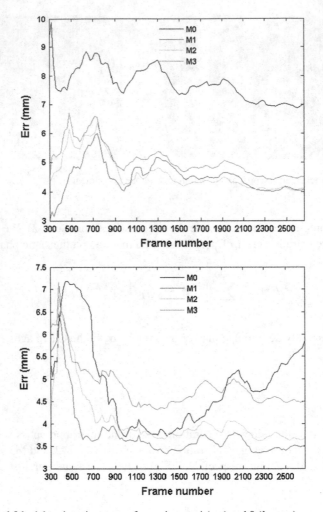

Fig. 5 Plotted fiducial registration error of experiments 4 (*top*) and 8 (*bottom*)

of the four methods evaluated by Experiments 4 and 8. Figure 6 investigates the distance between the sensor measurements and the bronchial centerlines. Figures 7 and 8 displays the sensor measurements that were transformed to CT using different matrices estimated by methods of M0, M1, and M2.

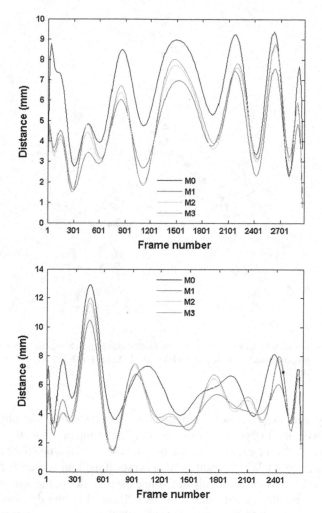

Fig. 6 Distance between sensor measurements and bronchial centerlines of experiments 7 (*top*) and 10 (*bottom*) were compared. Average distances of M0, M1, M2, and M3 were 6.1, 4.3, 4.5, and 4.6 mm, respectively

5 Discussion

In general, our proposed methods (M1, M2, and M3) to perform marker-free registration procedures can significantly reduce the fiducial registration error compared the previous method [8]; because our methods compute the position of the endoscope tip center based on sensor measurements to replace the direct position of EMT sensor measurements, enabling our algorithms to use points that are closest to the centerlines (Figs. 6, 7, and 8); we successfully released the assumption discussed above. The two-sensor-based method is possibly better than the three-sensor-based.

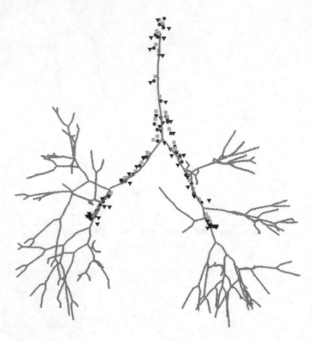

Fig. 7 Sensor measurements of experiment 1 were plotted along bronchial centerlines. Our selected points from our proposed methods of M1 and M2 (*red* O and *green* □) are closer to bronchial centerlines than M0 (*black* ∇)

Theoretically speaking, three points can accurately determine one and only one circle center. However, due to dynamic errors such as jitter jump or magnetic field distortion, it is possible for the excenters of the two-sensor-based method to be closer than the three-sensor-based. We may add another sensor (total four sensors) on the endoscope tip in order to more accurately determine the excenter of the four point plane. Moreover, our registration accuracy remains influenced by the dynamic magnetic field distortion of the EMT system that also has 0.88 mm static error. Also note that we here did not consider respiratory motion, which usually deteriorates the accuracy and will be evaluated on patient datasets or a dynamic phantom that can sumilate the breathig motion in the future.

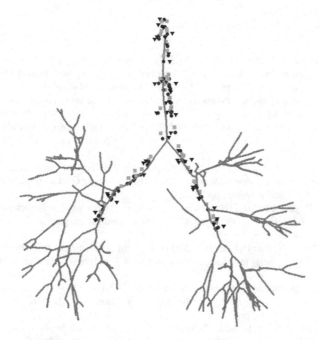

Fig. 8 Sensor measurements of experiment 3 were plotted along bronchial centerlines. Our selected points from our proposed methods of M1 and M2 (*red* O and *green* □) are closer to bronchial centerlines than M0 (*black* ∇)

6 Conclusions

This work proposed an improved fiducial-free registration approach for real-time and robust endoscope electromagnetic tracking and navigation. We introduced the endoscope tip center position to replace the sensor measurement position during optimization. We successfully tackled an assumption that an endoscope is operated along the hollow organ centerlines during endoscopic interventions. Our proposed method significantly reduced the fiducial registration error from at least 6.3 to 4.0 mm compared to previous methods. Future work includes improvement of endoscope electromagnetic tracking and patient data validation.

Acknowledgments This work was partly supported by the center of excellence project called the "Development of high-precision bedside devices for early metastatic cancer diagnosis and surgery" (01-D-D0806) funded by Aichi Prefecture, the JSPS Kakenhi "Modality-seamless navigation for endoscopic diagnosis and surgery assistance based on multi-modality image fusion" (25242047), and the "Computational anatomy for computer-aided diagnosis and therapy: frontiers of medical image sciences" (21103006) funded by a Grant-in-Aid for Scientific Research on Innovative Areas, MEXT, Japan.

References

1. Luo X, Feuerstein M, Deguchi D, Kitasaka T, Takabatake H, Mori K (2012) Development and comparison of new hybrid motion tracking for bronchoscopic navigation. MedIA 16(3):577–596
2. Gergel I, dos Santos TR, Tetzlaff R, Maier-Hein L, Meinzer H-P, Wegner I (2010) Particle filtering for respiratory motion compensation during navigated bronchoscopy. In: Wong KH, Miga, MI (eds) SPIE Medical Imaging 2010, California USA, vol 7625, pp 76250W
3. Soper TD, Haynor DR, Glenny RW, Seibel EJ (2010) In vivo validation of a hybrid tracking system for navigation of an ultrathin bronchoscope within peripheral airways. IEEE Trans Biomed Eng 57(3):736–745
4. Luo X, Kitasaka T, Mori K (2011) Bronchoscopy navigation beyond electromagnetic tracking systems: a novel bronchoscope tracking prototype. In: Fichtinger G, et al. (eds) MICCAI 2011, Part I, LNCS, Springer, vol 6891, pp 194–202
5. Cornish DC, Higgins WE (2012) Bronchoscopy guidance system based on bronchoscope-motion measurements. In: Holmes III DR, Wong KH (eds) SPIE Medical Imaging 2012, California USA, vol 8316, pp 83161G
6. Schwarz Y, Greif J, Becker HD, Ernst A, Mehta A (2006) Real-time electromagnetic navigation bronchoscopy to peripheral lung lesions using overlaid CT images: The first human study. Chest 129(4):988–994
7. Klein T, Traub J, Hautmann H, Ahmadian A, Navab N (2007) Fiducial-free registration procedure for navigated bronchoscopy. In: Ayache N, Ourselin S, Maeder A (eds) MICCAI 2007, Part I, LNCS, Springer, vol 4791, pp 475–482
8. Deguchi D, Feuerstein M, Kitasaka T, Suenaga Y, Ide I, Murase H, Imaizumi K, Hasegawa Y, Mori K (2012) Real-time marker-free patient registration for electromagnetic navigated bronchoscopy: a phantom study. Int J Comput Assist Radiol Surg 7(3):359–369

Evaluation of Image Guided Robot Assisted Surgical Training for Patient Specific Laparoscopic Surgery

Tao Yang, Kyaw Kyar Toe, Chin Boon Chng, Weimin Huang, Chee Kong Chui, Jiang Liu and Stephen K. Y. Chang

Abstract Image guided robot assisted surgical (IRAS) training was applied to train users in acquiring motor skills for laparoscopic surgery. Virtual surgery experiments were conducted to verify the effectiveness of this training method and compare with that of conventional training. The participants received image guided robot assisted training spent lesser time and shorter trajectory length in completing the same tasks when comparing with participants who were trained by conventional training method. Performance of the two groups of participants were also evaluated by a Hidden Markov Model which represents the surgeon's performance. The group

T. Yang (✉) · K. K. Toe · W. Huang
Neural and Biomedical Technology Department, Institute for Infocomm Research,
Singapore 138632, Singapore
e-mail: tyang@i2r.a-star.edu.sg

K. K. Toe
e-mail: kktoe@i2r.a-star.edu.sg

W. Huang
e-mail: wmhuang@i2r.a-star.edu.sg

T. Yang · C. B. Chng · C. K. Chui
Department of Mechanical Engineering, National University of Singapore,
Singapore 117575, Singapore
e-mail: mpeccb@nus.edu.sg

C. K. Chui
e-mail: mpecck@nus.edu.sg

J. Liu
Ocular Imaging Programme, Institute for Infocomm Research, Singapore 138632, Singapore
e-mail: jliu@i2r.a-star.edu.sg

S. K. Y. Chang
Department of Surgery, National University Hospital, Singapore 119074, Singapore
e-mail: cfscky@nus.edu.sg

J. M. R. S. Tavares et al. (eds.), *Bio-Imaging and Visualization for Patient-Customized Simulations*, Lecture Notes in Computational Vision and Biomechanics 13,
DOI: 10.1007/978-3-319-03590-1_7, © Springer International Publishing Switzerland 2014

receiving IRAS training achieved higher probability of observation sequences than that of the group receiving conventional training. This study suggests that the IRAS training method is effective in transferring motor skills from surgeon to other users.

1 Introduction

Laparoscopic surgery is a preferred surgical method for all technically possible cases. However due to the nature of laparoscopic surgery itself, physical and visual constraints such as work space limitations and hand-eye coordinations are imposed onto the surgeons [1]. Therefore, intensive training is required for medical residents to acquire the necessary skills and proficiency before they can operate on real patients. Although the skills can be developed in conventional operating room environments, costs and safety concerns with respect to practicing on patients limit on the amount of training attempts residents can experience. Numerous training equipments which allow medical residents to practice their laparoscopic skills are available commercially, ranging from box trainer to virtual reality training system [2]. However, these training equipment only provide a controlled environment to practice in. The users have to practice and hone their skills without guidance by themselves, or with guidance only with external supervision, such as experienced surgeons.

Physical guidance is an intuitive and effective method in training motor skills [3]. Physical guidance can be applied in laparoscopic surgical training as well. Experienced surgeons occasionally guide medical residents by holding their hands, or correcting their arm gestures in order to show the appropriate way of handling surgical instruments in a specific scenario. In our previous work, we proposed an Image Guided Robot Assisted surgical (IRAS) training system to record the movement of a surgical instrument in a virtual surgical operation and use the robotic technologies together with the recorded procedure to demonstrate and guide the trainees in honing their motor skills for laparoscopic surgery [4].

In this paper, we evaluate the effectiveness of the IRAS training system. Basic evaluation criteria, such as total task time, path length, path smoothness and traumas on the organs were applied by other researchers in evaluating virtual reality surgical simulators [5, 6] and robotic assisted surgery [7]. While these evaluation criteria provide information in overall performance, they hardly reflect how close the trainee's performance is to the experienced surgeon's performance, especially from medical staff's perspective. Another commonly used technique in evaluating surgical performance is the Hidden Markov Model (HMM). Researchers applied HMM technologies in evaluating the proficiency levels of the participants in using LapSim simulator for minimally invasive surgical training [8] and the proficiency levels of surgeons in using the Da Vinci surgical system [9].

The objective of this paper is to study the difference between the image guided robot assisted surgical (IRAS) training method and conventional training method in acquiring laparoscopic surgical skills. We applied HMM techniques to compare the performance of two groups of participants where one group of participants received the IRAS training and the other group of participants received their training by watching a video of virtual surgery. The remaining paper is organized as follows: Sect. 2 describes the surgical training system, surgical scenario and HMM evaluation method for this study. Section 3 explains our experiment method in detail. The performance of the participants is evaluated and discussed in Sect. 4. Finally, our work is concluded in Sect. 5.

2 Robotic Surgical Training Method

2.1 Surgical Simulation System

The IRAS training system consists of two modules, the robotic laparoscopic surgical trainer and the surgical simulation platform, as shown in Figs. 1 and 2. Both modules are connected by a dedicated Ethernet communication network.

The robotic laparoscopic surgical trainer serves as a human-machine interface in both processes of acquiring surgical procedure and providing guidance to the users [4]. The robot was designed to mimic the motion kinematics of the laparoscopic instruments in the real surgery [4]. Users can operate with the robotic handles (Fig. 2a), using them to perform a virtual surgery. The motion information of the robotic handles are sent to the surgical simulation platform to drive the virtual instruments and operate on the virtual organs. Motion trajectories of the robotic han-

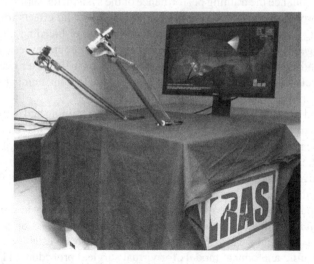

Fig. 1 Image guided robot assisted surgical (IRAS) simulation system for patient specific surgical training and surgical planning

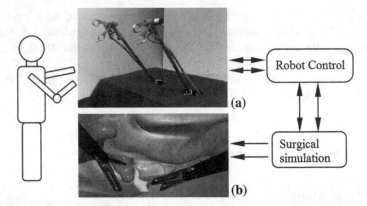

Fig. 2 IRAS simulation system diagram: robotic laparoscopic surgical trainer (**a**) and surgical simulation platform (**b**)

dles, virtual instruments and statues of the tool-tissue interaction are recorded for the purpose of training and analysis.

The surgical simulation platform comprises of patients virtual organs, a tool library of laparoscopic instruments and physics engines. The tool library contains common instruments required for laparoscopic surgery, such as forceps with different shapes and sizes, hook electrode, clip applicator and scissors. Tool-tissue interactions, organ deformation, tissue division and other activities executed during surgery are simulated in the surgical simulation platform.

In order to enhance the training performance of the system, the surgical simulation platform incorporates smoke, bleeding, perforation and audio effects for the operations involving hook electrodes and scissors. Activation of bleeding and perfusion effects is triggered by the collision of objects, angle and contact pressure between the tool tip and organ surface. A basic assessment is provided after every surgical simulation, including time spent, average velocity of the tool tip, number of bleeding sites and perforations that occurred.

A simulated surgical procedure can be reproduced for training and demonstration. Motion of the robotic handle and tool-tissue interaction can be replayed on the robot and the surgical simulation platform simultaneously. The user can hold on to the moving robotic handles while watching the simulated surgical procedure to appreciate the maneuvers conducted by the experienced surgeon. Motor skills training can be conducted through such a record and replay procedure.

The system is designed for patient specific laparoscopic surgery training and simulation in which a model of any patient can be generated based on CT data and configured for a virtual surgery [10]. A framework has been established to generate patient specific anatomical models for virtual surgical procedure [11]. Nineteen patients' abdominal CT images were segmented, analyzed and built as virtual patients for the laparoscopic cholecystectomy surgery. This allows medical residents to be exposed to a variety of surgical cases and provides them with a preview of any variation in anatomy before they start the surgery.

2.2 Surgical Scenario

A segment of the cholecystectomy surgical procedure is selected as the experimental scenario in the simulation. This segment begins with the liver and the gallbladder lifted up and exposed. A grasping forceps (Fig. 3a) is inserted from the left port to grasp the Hartman's pouch of the gallbladder and pull to stretch the cystic duct. A small hook electrode (Fig. 3a) is inserted from the right port to ablate the connective tissue and dissect the cystic duct. When the ablation process is completed, the instrument in the right port is changed to a curved forceps (Fig. 3b). This forceps is inserted between the cystic duct and the liver for inspection to ensure that all connective tissue has been fully ablated. Once complete, a clip applicator (Fig. 3c) is inserted from the right port to deploy three clips onto the cystic duct. While the clips can also be deployed on the cystic artery in real surgeries, the artery is not modeled in this scenario. After deployment of the clips, the instrument in the right port is

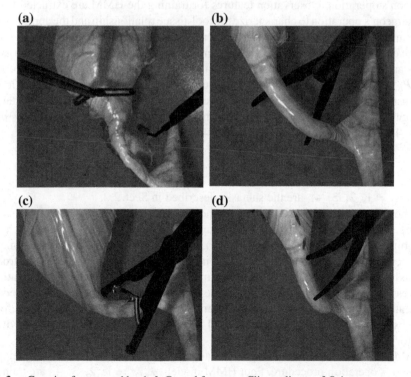

(a)   (b)

(c)   (d)

Fig. 3 **a** Grasping forceps and hook, **b** Curved forceps, **c** Clip applicator, **d** Scissors

changed to a laparoscopic scissors (Fig. 3d), and the cystic duct is divided. Two clips are left on the cystic duct to ensure that the cystic duct has been clamped securely.

During the entire virtual surgery, the main task of the instrument in the left port is to grab onto the gallbladder and stretch the cystic duct, providing room and allowing the instrument from right port with more access to carry out the procedure. The procedure described above was chosen as the evaluation procedure as it is a critical procedure in cholecystectomy surgery. Requirements from medical perspective such as the place of grabbing, the orientation of curved forceps, need to be taken into consideration while using each instrument. The entire series of tasks can be further divided into 4 subtasks based on the instrument in the right port as follows:

Subtask 1: ablation of the connective tissue and dissection of the cystic duct;

Subtask 2 : checking the clearance between the cystic duct and the liver;

Subtask 3 : deployment of three clips on the cystic duct;

Subtask 4 : division of the cystic duct.

2.3 Performance Modeling by HMM

The virtual surgery used for the IRAS training is recorded from an experienced surgeon's operation. Observation features for training the HMM are extracted from the surgeon's operation to characterize the tool-tissue relationship and the appropriate way in manipulating the surgical instruments. The observation features include the relative position of the left and right instruments to the specified points on the organ, P_{LO} and P_{RO}; the position and orientation of the left and right instruments' tip, P_L and P_R; the opened angle of surgical instrument's handle, α_L and α_R; the angle of the instrument's tip vector to the specific vectors on the organ, β_L and β_R; the status of footswitch, F_R; the vector from left instrument's tip to the right instrument's tip, P_{LR}. These features are illustrated in Fig. 4. It is expressed as

$$O_s = \{P_{LO} \quad P_{RO} \quad P_L \quad \alpha_L \quad P_R \quad \alpha_R \quad \beta_L \quad \beta_R \quad P_{LR}\}, \tag{1}$$

where $s = 1, 2, 3, 4$, are the subtasks described in Sect. 2.2.

These features are selected to capture the operation performed on the organ, such as the places where the instruments operate on, status of the instrument (such as grabbing, ablation, deploying and cutting), Relative position of the left instrument with respect to the right instrument and the instruments to organs. As a hook electrode is used in subtask 1, the angle of the instrument's handle has no effect to the ablation process. The signal from footswitch and the position of hook electrode can be used to indicate whether the user activates the ablation process at the right places. Therefore the observation feature α_R in expression (1) is replaced with the status of footswitch F_R for subtask 1 only.

HMM with full transition using Gaussian distribution is constructed to model the surgeon's operation procedure. Four HMM models, $\lambda_s, s = 1, 2, 3, 4$, are trained to represent the 4 subtasks. In order to construct HMM models that could adequately

(a)   (b)

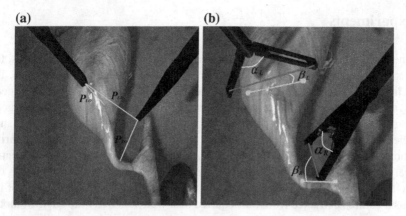

Fig. 4 Instruments' tip to the specified points on the organ, P_{LO} and P_{RO} ; relative position vector from the *left* instrument's tip to the *right* instrument's, P_{LR} ; angle between the instrument's tip vector and the specific vectors on the organ, β_L and β_R ; angle of the instrument handle opened, α_L and α_R , they are proportional to the angle of applicator's jaws formed

represent the surgeon's performance, cross validation is applied to determine the optimal number of states for the HMM models. Each HMM model is set with 3 states as illustrated in Fig. 5. The initial parameters are estimated by k-means classification method for the Gaussian distribution. The expectation maximization (EM) algorithm is applied to estimate the parameters of the HMM models [12].

The probability of observation sequence is used as a measure of the similarity of trainees' performance to the surgeon's performance. This similarity is measured in terms of the observation features described in expression (1). Observation sequences $O_{t,s}$ extracted from the 4 subtasks conducted by trainees are input into the respective HMM model to find out their probabilities. The probability of the observation sequence generated by the surgeon's HMM model is expressed as $P_{t,s}(O_{t,s}|\lambda_s)$, where s is the number of the subtask, t is the serial number of the trainee.

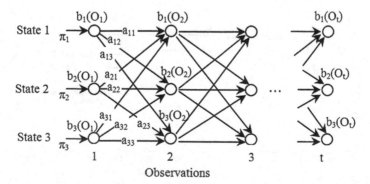

Fig. 5 3 states full transition Hidden Markov Model. π is the prior probability, a is the state transition matrix and b is the observation probability

3 Experiments

For the purpose of evaluating the difference between the two training methods, the effects of difficulty levels in the virtual surgery should be minimized. Hence, the experiment was conducted on the same patient's model. An experienced surgeon performed the procedure described in Sect. 2.2, a total of 10 times. The surgeon performed the virtual surgery with the same requirements as in real surgery, such as selecting the tissue grasping location, orientation of the instrument tip during ablation and visibility of the instrument tip for different instruments. The entire virtual surgical procedure was recorded, including the trajectory of instrument's tip, the relative position of the instruments' tip to the organ, and the deformation of the organs. Features extracted from the acquired data were taken to train a HMM model to serve as a reference model for comparison with the participants' performances. Fig. 6 shows the convergence of EM algorithm in training HMM models for the 4 subtasks. One of the acquired procedure was chosen by the surgeon to work as a guiding reference to train the participants in the experiment.

Twelve subjects, with an average age of 22.3 ± 3 years and no medical experiences participated in the study. They were randomly divided into two groups with 6 participants in each group, namely Group A and Group B. Since neither participant had medical background, they were first introduced with cholecystectomy and the function of each laparoscopic instruments as mentioned in Sect. 2.2. All participants were given 3 h each to familiarize themselves with the training system a day before the experiment. In order to obtain a sense of how the laparoscopic instruments worked and how to use the robotic system to perform virtual surgery, they practiced on pointing, grabbing, moving, clipping and dividing operations with the training system. After familiarization with the robotic system, the task was then described to all participants.

Participants in Group A underwent the image guided robot assisted training using the system as shown in Fig. 1. The handles of the robotic system moved along the

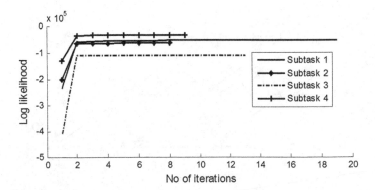

Fig. 6 Convergence of log likelihood for each subtask in parameter estimation process

recorded trajectories of the experienced surgeon while the virtual surgical scene corresponding to the movement of surgical instruments and tool-tissue interaction was also replayed on a wide screen monitor simultaneously. Participants were required to place their hands on the robotic handles to experience the motion of the surgical instrument while watching the surgical simulation scene at the same time. Conversely, the participants in Group B received their training by watching a video of the virtual surgery. All participants were informed to concentrate on how the instruments were manipulated, including relative position to the organ, orientation of the instrument's tip and angle of the instrument's handle opened. The simulated surgical procedures showed to both Group A and B were identical.

All participants were required to experience one session of training, followed by one session of practice on the virtual patient. This training and practice cycle was repeated 5 times. Upon completion of the 5 cycles of training and practice sessions, all participants were required to complete 10 tests of the entire task. There were practices and 120 tests in total. All participants went through the 5 cycles of training and practice sessions, concluding with the test session.

4 Performance Analysis and Discussions

Average task time utilized, trajectory length for left and right instruments were calculated to evaluate the participants' overall performance on the task. The overall performance of the surgeon was also evaluated by these basic evaluation criteria and they are shown in Table 1. The participants in Group B took longer task time and utilized longer trajectory length to complete the task as compare to Group A. The participants from Group B may have behaved more hesitant in performing the tasks; they may have exercised more trial-and-error attempts while navigating the instrument to approach the organ due to the constraints in depth perception [13]. Similarly, due to the limited depth information inherently obtainable from watching training videos, the participants of Group B may have spent more time establishing their sense of depth during the practice and test sessions, resulting in the utilization of longer time and trajectory length. In contrast, Table 1 shows that the task time and trajectory length for participants in Group A to complete the tasks is closer to the surgeon's performance. This might suggest that the motor skills required to perform the tasks have been demonstrated and transferred from the surgeon to the participants.

Table 1 Surgeon and participants' performance evaluated by average task time, trajectory length of the left and right instruments

	Participants	Time (s)	Left (mm)	Right (mm)
	Surgeon	239.5 ± 38	530.1 ± 184.4	1512.0 ± 144.2
Test session	Group A	246.7 ± 70.9	579.8 ± 275.4	1578.3 ± 369.0
	Group B	268.4 ± 149.5	978.7 ± 861.4	1850.6 ± 824.0
	p value	0.18	<0.001	0.011

Applying T-test on Group A and B, we can notice that the difference between both groups in trajectory length is statistically significant ($p < 0.05$). On the other hand, task time may not be an effective evaluation criteria ($p > 0.05$) to identify the difference between both group's performances.

Observation sequences from participants' 10 test sessions were fed to the surgeon's HMM model to obtain the probabilities of observation sequences. They were obtained using forward-backward algorithm [12] and expressed in log likelihood. The mean log likelihood of two group's each test session for each subtask are shown in Fig. 7. Participants from Group A generally produced higher log likelihood and smaller standard deviation than Group B in all 4 subtasks. Although Fig. 7. shows that Group A's performance is closer to the surgeon's model than Group B, more tests are required to confirm the results statistically.

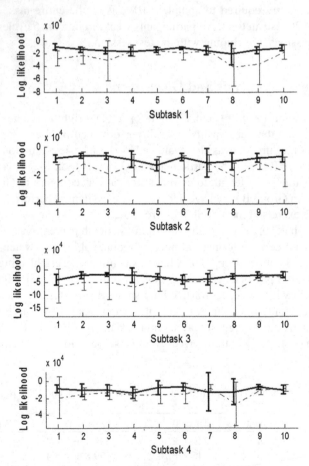

Fig. 7 Mean log likelihood and standard deviation of each group of participants at each test session. *Dark solid lines* represent Group A, *dash lines* represent Group B, *vertical bars* represent the standard deviation of the likelihood for each test session

Table 2 Percentages of the observation sequences from Group A and ranked at top N of the 120 observation sequences (N = 20, 40, 60)

	Top 20 (%)	Top 40 (%)	Top 60 (%)
Subtask 1	65.0	67.5	65.0
Subtask 2	90.0	77.5	70.0
Subtask 3	60.0	52.5	53.3
Subtask 4	70.0	72.5	58.3

The 120 probabilities of observation sequences generated by the surgeon's HMM model for both group and each subtask were ranked. Percentages of the observation sequences from Group A and ranked at top 20, 40 and 60 of the 120 sets of observation sequence are listed in Table 2. Based on the results, Group A obtained the majority of top 20, 40 and 60 of the 120 sets of observation sequences of all 4 subtasks. This suggests that the participants from Group A tried to execute their virtual surgery in a similar way to the surgeon. The performance of Group A is closer to the surgeon's performance in terms of the observation features.

5 Conclusion

There are numerous training equipments and methods to assist surgeons in acquiring motor skills required for laparoscopic surgery. In this paper, we conducted experiments on IRAS training system to compare the efficiency between image guided robot assisted training method and conventional training method. During the test session, participants who received IRAS training took lesser task time and shorter trajectory length to complete the tasks. The difference in utilized trajectory length between the two groups has been found to be statistically significant. We also applied HMM to characterize and compare the performance of participants and the surgeon. Group A which received image guided robot assisted training produced higher average probability of observation sequence as compared to Group B. The results suggests that the IRAS training system is more effective in transferring motor skills to the user than that of the conventional training method. As the IRAS training system is capable in simulating patient specific surgical scenario, this allows the surgeon to conduct patient specific medical education, especially for cases involving rare anatomies and/or pathologies. In this study, relatively simple tasks were used for the evaluation. More complicated scenarios can be constructed for future studies. Currently, we are conducting another study involving senior medical students and surgical training using animals.

Acknowledgments This work is partially supported by research grant BEP 102 148 0009, Image-guided Robotic Assisted Surgical Training from the Agency for Science, Technology and Research, Singapore. We would like to express our thanks to Ms Zhang Zhuo for her valuable assistance in statistical analysis.

References

1. Heemskerk J et al (2006) Advantages of advanced laparoscopic systems. Surg Endosc 20(5):730–3
2. Sutherland LM et al (2006) Surgical simulation: a systematic review. Ann Surg 243(3):291–300
3. Wulf G, Shea CH, Whitacre CA (1998) Physical-guidance benefits in learning a Complex motor skill. J Mot Behav 30:367–380
4. Yang T, et al (2012) Mechanism of a learning robot manipulator for laparoscopic surgical training. Intell Auton Syst 12:17–26
5. Woodrum DT et al (2006) Construct validity of the LapSim laparoscopic surgical simulator. Am J Surg 191(1):28–32
6. Sanchez-Peralta LF et al (2012) Learning curves of basic laparoscopic psychomotor skills in SINERGIA VR simulator. Int J Comput Assist Radiol Surg 7(6):881–889
7. Kho RM (2011) Comparison of robotic-assisted laparoscopy versus conventional laparoscopy on skill acquisition and performance. Clin Obstet Gynecol 54(3):376–81
8. Megali G et al (2006) Modelling and evaluation of surgical performance using hidden Markov models. IEEE Trans Biomed Eng 53(10):1911–1919
9. Reiley CE, Plaku E, Hager GD (2010) Motion generation of robotic surgical tasks: learning from expert demonstrations. In: 2010 Annual International Conference of the IEEE Engineering in Medicine and Biology Society (EMBC), 2010
10. Zhou J, et al (2010) Segmentation of gallbladder from CT images for a surgical training system. In: 2010 3rd International Conference on Biomedical Engineering and Informatics (BMEI), 2010
11. Law GH, Eng M, Lim CW, Su Y, Huang W, Zhou J, Liu J, Zhang J, Yang T, Chui CK, Chang S (2011) Rapid generation of patient-specific anatomical models for usage in virtual environment. Comput Aided Des Appl 8(6):927–938
12. Rabiner L, Juang B (1986) An introduction to hidden Markov models. IEEE ASSP Mag 3(1):4–16
13. Vassiliou MC et al (2005) A global assessment tool for evaluation of intraoperative laparoscopic skills. Am J Surg 190(1):107–13

Proxemics Measurement During Social Anxiety Disorder Therapy Using a RGBD Sensors Network

Julien Leroy, François Rocca and Bernard Gosselin

Abstract In this paper, we focus on the development of a new ecological methodology to study proxemics behaviors. We based our approach on a network of RGBD cameras, calibrated together. The use of this type of sensors lets us build a 3D multiview recording installation working in various natural settings. The skeleton tracking functionalities, provided by the multiple 3D data, are a useful tool to make proxemics observation and automatically code these non-verbal cues. Our goal is to propose a new approach to study proxemics behaviors of patients suffering from social anxiety disorder to improve observation capabilities of the therapist with an unobtrusive, ecological and precise measurement system.

1 Introduction

The study of your spatial behavior can reveal lot of information about you. Indeed, even if people feel free to move, many rules unconsciously shape their evolution, their use of space. Speed, direction or trajectory are controlled and comply with various patterns constrained by social mechanisms [17]. Proxemics is a domain of research that investigates the way people use and organize physical space around them while interacting with others. E. T. Hall, an American anthropologist, introduced for the first time this concept in his studies about the human behavior in public space [12] and defined it as

J. Leroy (✉) · F. Rocca · B. Gosselin
TCTS Lab, University Of Mons, 31 Boulevard Dolez, 7000 Mons, Belgium
e-mail: julien.leroy@umons.ac.be

F. Rocca
e-mail: francois.rocca@umons.ac.be

B. Gosselin
e-mail: bernard.gosselin@umons.ac.be

J. M. R. S. Tavares et al. (eds.), *Bio-Imaging and Visualization for Patient-Customized Simulations*, Lecture Notes in Computational Vision and Biomechanics 13, DOI: 10.1007/978-3-319-03590-1_8, © Springer International Publishing Switzerland 2014

[...] the study of man's transactions as he perceives and use intimate, personal, social and public space in various settings [...].

Since this first development, much research has been conducted in the field of psychology and social science related to the concept of proxemics and one of its most important aspects: the interpersonal distances. The study of social spaces and proxemics can obviously lead to a better understanding of social mechanisms and context but also to developments in many areas such as robotics, human-computer interactions, teaching methodologies, etc. This paper focus on the development of a new methodology to study proxemics behaviors that try to solve some of the main issues raised by ethologists:

1. Unobtrusive means and ecological conditions.
2. Easy setting in various environments.
3. Precise measurements.
4. Simplify and accelerate experiments.

Our solution is based on a framework using multiple RGB-Depth(RGB-D) cameras. This choice, lets us create large 3D observation scene coupled with possibilities of users and skeleton tracking to extract non-verbal cues linked to proxemics behaviors. The main element of our system is a network of RGB-D cameras calibrated together to realize ecological recordings of the interactions. On these recordings, we apply skeleton tracking algorithm to automatically extract information about the behaviors that can be used by a psychologist to code the interaction like proposed by [13]. This research and developments take place in a long-term study of proxemics behaviors in social anxiety disorder (DSM-IV 300.23) [4], also known as social phobia. Our goal, with this new methodology, is to create a computer vision tool to assist and help the psychologist in the treatment of patients suffering of this type of disorder. Firstly, by giving an interactive visualization of proxemics cues to the patient and his therapist, to help the analysis of the interaction by modeling interpersonal distances. Secondly, to precisely record the spatial behavior of patients through time and see if these proxemics information can be used as indicators of the patient's progress through his therapy.

This chaper is organized as follows. Section 2 introduces the main concepts of proxemics. Section 3 presents a state-of-the-art of the methodologies and settings use to study proxemics behaviors. Section 4 details our system and how we tried to solve the main problems in ethological experiment. Section 5 reports some experiments on which we apply our methodology and Sect. 6 draws some conclusions.

2 Proxemics Fundamentals

Proxemics is the study of how man unconsciously organize, share, use physical space and the underlying meaning of these spatial behaviors both on social interactions and human psyche. The most important aspect of proxemics behaviors is probably the notion of interpersonal distances, these areas unconsciously established by people between them. The first part of this section will give some enlightenment about this social signal. The second part will be dedicated to detail some factors that can be used to caracterize proxemics interactions and we want to put in evidence with our methodology.

2.1 Interpersonal Distances

People create unconscious territories around them, which define and determine the interactions they can have with other individuals. Those territories are like some invisible bubbles surrounding them and keeping them far from each other, unless space has some physical constraints (small room, crowded environment...). Interpersonal distances are a form of non-verbal communication between two or more persons defined by the social relationship they have. In a way, the measure of these distances is a clue that can tell us how people know each other. E.T.Hall has proposed a first model, based on the study of the spatial behavior of the American middle class people, that divides the space around a person in four distinct regions Fig. 1:

1. Intimate distance (0–45 cm): a really close space with high probability of physical contact. It's a distance for touching, whispering or embracing someone. It indicates a close relationship like with lovers or children.
2. Personal distance (45 cm–1.2 m): distance for interacting with relatives like family members or good friends. Unrequested penetration of this space will provoke discomfort, defensive postures and even avoidance behaviors.

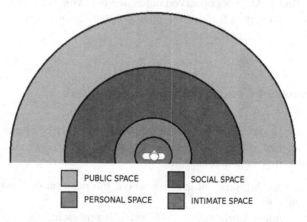

PUBLIC SPACE   SOCIAL SPACE

PERSONAL SPACE   INTIMATE SPACE

Fig. 1 Definition of Hall's interpersonal space model. The space around people is divided in four territories: the intimate space, the personal space, the social space and the public space

3. Social distance (1.2–3.5 m): distance for more formal or impersonal interactions. It's the distance you naturally pose when you meet stranger and establish a communication process with them.
4. Public distance (3.5–infinity): distance for mass meeting, lecture hall or interactions with important personalities.

In fact, many parameters are influencing the shape and size of our personal spaces. In his work, he also showed the cultural differences in the use of space and the impact this could have on the size of interpersonal distances. It classifies populations into two groups: contact and non-contact cultures. For instance, for Japanese people, a non-contact culture, the model should have larger separation distances, which would be the opposite for an Arab or Latin population.

People update, control and adjust these spaces continuously. Obviously social spaces are much more complex social mechanisms and depend on many parameters. They continuously evolve and adapt to people circumstances. They should be seen as dynamic and elastic territories varying with lot of parameters like: culture, sex, age, gender, size, social position, relationship or physical appearance. Social sciences have already explored a lot this subject and showed the importance of this concept for explaining how people behave but also in some medical case like with schizophrenic patients [19]. Many behavioral experiments have shown the importance and impact that these distances could have on our actions. An example is the unauthorized penetration of these territories that will cause a feeling of discomfort for people. This can lead to an aggressive response of the subject who may feel oppressed by the presence of the intruder. In the case of social anxious patients, this kind of behavior is often accentuated. The main feature that appeard about their proxemics behavior is a tendancy to have a bigger personal space, a larger confort zone that keeps them away from social interraction but also generates a high level of anxiety when people invade their territory. An other observed defensive behavior is the body orientation where they try to not stay in front of the others. Situation understood like a miss of implication in the social interaction.

2.2 Visual Cues to Code Proxemics Interactions

E. T. Hall proposed a system to code proxemic behaviors [13] like a function of height indicators. In our methodology, we were only interested by some visual indicators that we wanted to highlight and measure:

1. Postural identifer. Minimal information about the position of a subject: prone, sitting or standing.
2. Sociofugal–sociopetal orientation (SPF axis). It represents the spatial position, orientation that pushes or pulls people to interact together. It's a function of the bodies' orientation, shoulders' position between each person. Hall proposed to code this on a height positions compass. Two subjects face to face would be

maximum sociopetality and back to back, maximum sociofugality with intermediate possibilities.
3. Vision. Here is the gaze orientation that is use like an factor of involvement. Hall
   propose three zones base of the anatomy of the retina: fovea (direct gaze, 12°
   horizontal visual angle), macula (20°), peripheral vision (up to 180°).

3 Proxemics Measurement Systems: State-of-the-Art

In psychology, to conduct experiments on variations of interpersonal distances and
proxemics behaviors, three types of methodologies are used:

1. The projective method that pushes subjects to imagine a scene and represent how
   themselves or others react spatially to the scenario. We usually resort to the use of
   drawing or dolls. It was showed that this method could be regarded as unreliable,
   because it requires significant capacity for reflection. The subject need to project
   himself in the scene and mentally represent himself having a social interaction.
   This method allows to cover a large number of scenario but skews the observations
   that we could get [14].
2. The laboratory method that aims to produce a spatial scenario, like a handshake,
   in a controlled environment. The subjects are often aware of participating in an
   experiment, which can cause variations in the perception of the environment and
   thus truncate the action. This is the classical setting use by psychologists.
3. The observation method of collecting data by studying the interaction between
   people in their natural environment, using measurement techniques causing as little interference as possible. It is obvious this method is the most difficult to achieve
   since it requires precise measurement systems that can operate independently of
   the environment.

Until recently, measurements on proxemics behaviors were performed and coded
manually. Some resort to the use of video recordings using special rooms with for
example a floor grid [16]. This method lets them measure, a posteriori, interpersonal
distances and code proxemics behaviors but often with bias due to unnatural settings
and the conditions of the experimentation. More recently, an approach using virtual
reality appeared [21]. This method gives good results because people tend to behave
the same way in virtual world and in the real world [10]. As it is based on projection
and an heavy equipment is often installed on the patient, it is not obvious that they
can be considered ecological measurement. To our knowledge, few computer vision
systems have been designed to help solve these issues. [3] and [6] proposed two
solutions using cameras in a bird-eye setting. This is an interesting solution but
difficult to apply in various environment like a classroom or a meeting room.

4 Our Approach for Analysing Proxemics Interactions Based on Multiple RGB-D Sensors

Our system is divided into recording units, each consisting of a computer, connected to one or two RGB-D cameras. To obtain a 3D multi-view system, Fig. 2, that lets us observe behavioral scenes, each camera must be calibrated in space but also in time to avoid delay when we merge the different recordings. The spatial calibration can be performed in various ways: by manually manipulating point clouds or by using a SLAM (Simultaneous Localisation And Mapping) approach that allows us to know at any moment the position of the sensor. The actual prototype employs Kinect or Asus Xtion sensors using the OpenNI library to access the cameras data and to track users [20]. We record at 20 frames per second, with a VGA resolution (640 × 480 pixels) on each sensor. The sensor has a horizontal field of view of 57 and the depth range is between 1 and 4 m. Beyond this limit, an important decrease of accuracy appeared, as detailed in [11]. This depth limitation reinforces the idea of sing a sensor network to cover a wide area such as room dedicated to group therapy.

First, we present our calibration method to make the system adaptable to many situations. Second, we present the structure of our camera network to control all the units. Third, we present the extracted data we use to characterize proxemics behaviors.

4.1 Sensors Calibration

To enable our system to be used in a wide range of situations and to make the positionning step simple as possible, two approaches are proposed to calibrate each sensors by taking advantage of the color and depth information.

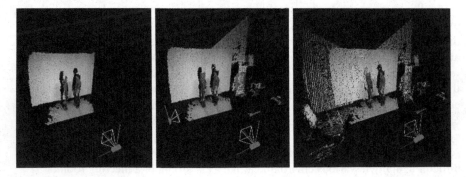

Fig. 2 Example of 3D multiview of the same proxemic scene with one, two and three calibrated sensors

1. Manual calibration: using clouds coming from already positioned sensors, we manualy manipulate the transformation matrix $[R|t]$ (rotation and translation) to stich the selected clouds and obtained their relative position in the 3D space.
2. SLAM calibration: a RGB-D registration algorithm is used, based on [15], and works in three steps: first, we calculate SIFT features on two consecutive images and then seek possible matches; second using RANSAC [9], we get a first estimation of the transformation between the two consecutive feature clouds; third, we apply an iterative closest point algorithm (ICP) [22] between the resulting point clouds to refine the transformation. This method, see Fig. 3, lets us freely move by hand a camera, knowing at each instant its position in space. Once each camera was positioned in this way, we know their position in space relative to a master camera which serves as a world reference.

4.2 Network Infrastructure

The cameras network operates with a master–slave architecture on a LAN network, Fig. 4. Each recording unit is a slave waiting UDP command from an distant master. The master is used to send a startup message on the network to initialize the recording. During the recording, a log file is created containing the timestamp of each saved frame. With this method, records can be resynchronized if it's necessary.

4.3 Data Extraction and Analysis

On each record is applied a skeleton tracking algorithm [5, 20]. Then, knowing the camera positions, all the skeletons are remapped in the same world coordinate frame. In the case where a user would have several skeletons due to overlapping areas, they can be merge by measuring the distance between similar joints. With the resulting

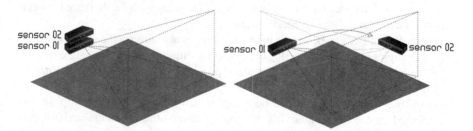

Fig. 3 Example of calibration between two sensors. A first camera is set then based on its initial view and point cloud, the second is moved to its final position. At each moment, we know the camera position in space with the RGBD SLAM algorithm

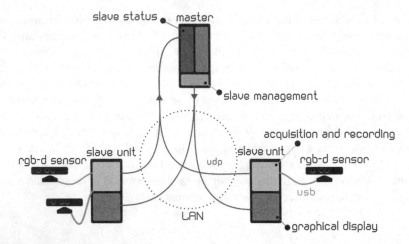

Fig. 4 Network infrastructure. One or two sensors can be connected to a slave unit. Record commands are send by a master unit

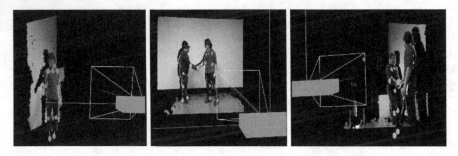

Fig. 5 Skeleton tracking applied on each view. These data are use to measure proxemics information like interpersonal distances or SPF orientation

multiview skeleton 3D data, Fig. 5, we can automatically process some proxemics information:

1. Interpersonal distances: they can be measure classicaly with the distance between users' centroids or head-to-head distances.
2. Postural identifier can be obtain with geometric constrains on the skeleton. Measuring angles produced by the legs can detect a sitting position. The angle formed by the head-torso line and the floor plane provides an estimate of the inclination of the upper body.
3. Sociofugal–socialpetal axis can be compute using the 3D shoulders' positions projected on the floor plane. It's the angle between the shoulders' axis of two interacting people.
4. Vision factor. To our knowledge, it is not possible to access the orientation of a person's eyes with RGB-D sensor in our operating conditions. This is mainly due to a too large distance between the sensor and the user and the freedom of

movement we want to give to the patients. The gaze normally consists of two components: it is a combination of both the direction of the eyes and the pose of the head. But as we can't access the eyes, one of the hypotheses on which we rely is that the gaze of a person is considered to be similar to the direction of his head. As stated in [18],

[...] Head pose estimation is intrinsically linked with visuel gaze estimation ... By itself, head pose provides a coarse indication of gaze that can be estimated in situations when the eyes of a person are not visible [...].

Several studies rely and validate this hypothesis as shown in [1]. The method used is based on the approach developed in [7, 8] and implemented in the PCL library [2]. This allows us to simultaneously detect faces but also to estimate their orientations on the depth map. The actual system needs a dedicated sensor close to the user like in Fig. 6.

5 Experiment and Discussion

We tested our system in the context of behavioral group therapy of patients suffering from social anxiety disorder. The goal was to use it to film exercises already integrated into therapy and to discuss what additional possibilities of measurement and analysis our system could provide. The system consisted of two recording units. Two cameras were sufficient to cover the entire area where took place the therapy sessions. These group therapy sessions are dedicated to the understanding of non-verbal communication and the importance it can have in social interactions. They aim to provoke awareness in patients about this form of language and the problems that can

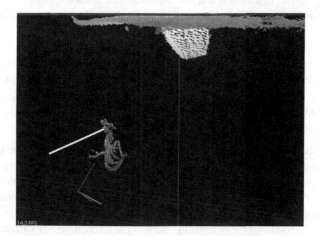

Fig. 6 Example of estimating the orientation of the head of a subject with a dedicated sensor positioned in proximity, in this case, the sensor was positioned between subjects at the knees level

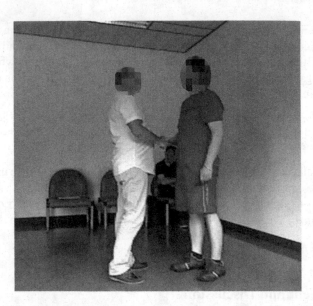

Fig. 7 Patient H1 (*white*), a meeting simulation. It is interesting in this case to observe the proximity of the two subjects, despite their stature and the little knowledge they have of each other. This proximity will result in H2 (*red*) several escape movements

affect it. Typically with such patients, it is the situations of discomfort and escape behaviors due to the proximity of others that are addressed. The recorded sessions dealt with territoriality, management of personal space and the physicality of the patient during dyadic interaction. Two exercises are performed by the therapist:

- *the meeting* He asked two patients to simulate a meeting, typically a handshake, followed by a brief discussion of a few minutes. The aim is to observe the evolution over time of the spatial behavior and gestures as well as the involvement in the discussion.
- *the search of the personal space* This exercise is dedicated to the search of his comfort zone to interact with someone. He asked a patient to stand still back to a wall (to limit the escape behavior), then a second participant must move forward and find the most comfortable to begin a discussion, then the roles are reversed distance. The distances of the two patients are compared and lead a discussion about their feelings during the experiment.

The first observation made on the videos is the inability of the practitioner to detect and manage all behavioral signs shown. Indeed, by the time constraints, he is obliged to perform the exercises simultaneously with several groups of patients. It is therefore difficult for him to fully concentrate on the interactions and raise the indices as we can do with the video. The second observation is that patients tend to distort the observations by "cheating" during the exercises. Six different patients were registered, four men and two women, for a total of 8 different dyadic groups. For each group, three exercises were filmed. The sessions were recorded twice: first at the

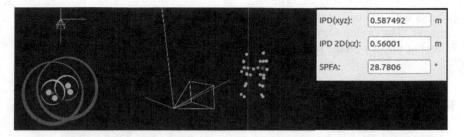

Fig. 8 Visualisation of the proxemics interaction 3D data extracted from Fig. 7. *Left*, the *top view* of the interaction, with in red the shoulders, in blue the body center and a representation of Hall's personal and intimate space. Center, a side view of the extracted skeletons. *Right*, measurement of proxemics information (interpersonal distance and shoulders angle). What can be observed about the patients' behavior is that they are really close to each other. Their body centers are at the limit of the intimate space, considering their body shape we can consider that they invade this territory. Which later induce an escape mechanism in one of the subjects

beginning of therapy and the second at the end (4 months with a weekly meeting). The objective of this double standard was to see if it was possible to measure behavioral changes in patients and the impact of therapy could have on them. We present below an example studied with our system. The most interesting patient, in a proxemics perspective, was a man of more than forty years (H1) presented by the therapist as having little presence and suffering from a lack of recognition towards others Fig. 7. The patient describes himself as "invisible". Its spatial behavior has the distinction of being invasive, without taking into account the behavioral response of others. For the therapist, it is the result of an affirmation need and an excessive difficulty in reading the nonverbal behavior of other participants. In our signals, (Fig. 8) it is denoted by:

- an personal space invasion of the other which also causes several escape
- almost no gesture.

At the end of therapy, his behavior has changed, his interpersonal distance increased (11 %), approaching the average personal space distance, causing less discomfort with his partner. For other patients, the behavior is more classic with a tendency to approach the others, sticking to the model, as patients are much more familiar. These encouraging results suggest that it should be possible to quantify the impact that therapy could have in a proxemics view point.

6 Conclusion

In this paper, we propose a new methodology to study proxemics behaviors and the preliminary results we obtained by testing the system in the case of social anxiety disorder therapy. The use of multiple RGBD cameras and the underlying tracking possibilities lets the experiment be natural, unobstrusive and precise. This should lead to good ecological data. The accuracy of our methodology makes it easy to identify patients with spatial behavior disorders but also to raise events that can escape the therapist. The preliminary results seem to show that it is possible to measure the impact of therapy on the patient behavior.

References

1. Abe K, Makikawa M (2010) Spatial setting of visual attention and its appearance in head-movement. IFMBE Proc 25(4):1063–1066
2. Aldoma A (2012) 3d face detection and pose estimation in pcl. Mach Learn 45(1):5–32
3. Amaoka T, Laga H (2010) Personal space modeling for human-computer interaction. In: Computing ICEC 2009, vol 5709, pp 60–72. http://www.springerlink.com/index/j24l366337456862.pdf
4. Association AP (2000) Diagnostic and statistical manual of mental disorders, 4th edn, Text Revision (DSM-IV-TR), 4th edn. American Psychiatric Association. http://www.worldcat.org/isbn/0890420254
5. Buys K, Cagniart C, Bashkeev A, Pantofaru C (2013) Detecting people and their poses using PointCloud Library. PCL (2012). Last viewed 26–07-2013 12:00
6. Cristani M, Paggetti G, Vinciarelli A, Bazzani L, Menegaz G, Murino V (2011) Towards computational proxemics: inferring social relations from interpersonal distances. Context 290–297. http://eprints.gla.ac.uk/58725/
7. Fanelli G, Dantone M, Gall J, Fossati A, Gool L (2013) Random forests for real time 3d face analysis. Int J Comput Vision 101:437–458. doi:10.1007/s11263-012-0549-0, http://dx.doi.org/10.1007/s11263-012-0549-0
8. Fanelli G, Weise T, Gall J, Gool LV (2011) Real time head pose estimation from consumer depth cameras. In: Proceedings of the 33rd international conference on Pattern recognition, DAGM'11, pp. 101–110. Springer-Verlag, Berlin, Heidelberg. http://dl.acm.org/citation.cfm?id=2039976.2039988
9. Fischler MA, Bolles, R.C.: Random sample consensus: a paradigm for model fitting with applications to image analysis and automated cartography. Commun ACM 24(6):381–395. doi:10.1145/358669.358692, http://portal.acm.org/citation.cfm?doid=358669.358692
10. Friedman D, Steed A, Slater M (2007) Spatial social behavior in second life. Intell Virtual Agents 4722(1997):252–263. http://discovery.ucl.ac.uk/190177/
11. Gonzalez-Jorge H, Riveiro B, Vazquez-Fernandez E, Martnez-Snchez J, Arias P (2013) Metrological evaluation of microsoft kinect and asus xtion sensors. Measurement 46(6):1800–1806 (2013). http://dx.doi.org/10.1016/j.measurement.2013.01.011, http://www.sciencedirect.com/science/article/pii/S0263224113000262
12. Hall ET (1996) The Hidden Dimension, vol 6. Doubleday. http://www.lavoisier.fr/notice/frPWOXLKSAOAWS2O.html
13. Hall ET (1963) A system for notation of proxemic behavior. Am Anthropologist 65:1003–1026
14. Hayduk LA (1983) Personal space: where we now stand. Psychol Bull 94(2):293–335. doi:10.1037//0033-2909.94.2.293, http://content.apa.org/journals/bul/94/2/293
15. Henry P, Krainin M, Herbst E, Ren X, Fox D (2010) RGB-D mapping : using depth cameras for dense 3D modeling of indoor environments. Work 1(c):9–10. http://ils.intel-research.net/uploads/papers/3d-mapping-iser-10-final.pdf
16. Ickinger WJ (1994) A study on simulation of proxemic behavior. Methodology 23:1–17
17. Murino V, Cristani M, Vinciarelli A (2010) Socially intelligent surveillance and monitoring: analysing social dimensions of physical space. Science 51–58. http://eprints.gla.ac.uk/40297/
18. Murphy-Chutorian E, Trivedi MM (2009) Head pose estimation in computer vision: a survey. IEEE Trans Pattern Anal Mach Intell 31(4):607–26. doi:10.1109/TPAMI.2008.106, http://www.ncbi.nlm.nih.gov/pubmed/19229078

19. Nechamkin Y, Salganik I, Modai I, Ponizovsky AM (2003) Interpersonal distance in schizophrenic patients: relationship to negative syndrome. Int J Soc Psychiatry 49(3):166–174.http://isp.sagepub.com/cgi/doi/10.1177/00207640030493002
20. OpenNI organization: OpenNI Programmer Guide (2010). http://www.openni.org/documentation Last viewed 17–03-2012 12:22
21. Wieser MJ, Pauli P, Grosseibl M, Molzow I, Mühlberger A (2010) Virtual social interactions in social anxiety-the impact of sex, gaze, and interpersonal distance. Cyberpsychology Behav Soc Networking 13(5):547–554 (2010). http://www.ncbi.nlm.nih.gov/pubmed/20950179
22. Zhang Z (1994) Iterative point matching for registration of free-form curves and surfaces. Int J Comput Vision 13(2):119–152 (1994). doi:10.1007/BF01427149, http://www.springerlink.com/index/10.1007/BF01427149

How Do Sex, Age, and Osteoarthritis Affect Cartilage Thickness at the Thumb Carpometacarpal Joint? Insights from Subject-Specific Cartilage Modeling

Eni Halilaj, David H. Laidlaw, Douglas C. Moore and Joseph J. Crisco

Abstract Studying the morphology of the thumb carpometacarpal (CMC) joint cartilage in both health and disease is warranted by the high incidence of CMC osteoarthritis (OA), especially in women; however, quantifying CMC cartilage variation *in vivo* remains challenging with current modalities. We used a subject-specific cartilage model that is based on joint space volume computations from sequential CT scans to find that cartilage thickness does not differ with sex and age, but that it does with early signs of OA. These findings advance the general understanding of CMC joint mechanics and OA pathogenesis by verifying that metabolic or genetic differences, under the influence of mechanical loading, rather than mechanical factors alone, are implicated in the pathoetiology of CMC OA. This model may be used to study cartilage degradation *in vivo*, may be incorporated into subject-specific mechanical simulations, and may have clinical applications for OA staging if combined with dynamic volume CT.

E. Halilaj (✉) · J. J. Crisco
Center for Biomedical Engineering, Brown University, Providence, RI, USA
e-mail: eni_halilaj@brown.edu

J. J. Crisco
e-mail: joseph_crisco@brown.edu

D. H. Laidlaw
Department of Computer Science, Brown University, Providence, RI, USA
e-mail: david_laidlaw@brown.edu

D. C. Moore · J. J. Crisco
Department of Orthopaedics, Warren Alpert Medical School of Brown University,
Providence, RI, USA
e-mail: douglas_moore@brown.edu

J. M. R. S. Tavares et al. (eds.), *Bio-Imaging and Visualization for Patient-Customized Simulations*, Lecture Notes in Computational Vision and Biomechanics 13, DOI: 10.1007/978-3-319-03590-1_9, © Springer International Publishing Switzerland 2014

1 Introduction

Osteoarthritis of the carpometacarpal (CMC) joint is a common and disabling disease with biological and mechanical factors implicated in its pathogenesis, but of unknown etiology and limited understanding of both microscopic and macroscopic mediators. The CMC joint is located at the base of the thumb (Fig. 1a) and is responsible for much of the dexterity of the human hand because of the flexibility of its articular geometry. Due to the pain and inflammation associated with it, CMC OA can significantly affect quality of life. The higher prevalence of CMC OA in women compared to men [1] and the increasing risk with age raise both biological and mechanical questions about potential differences with sex, age, and disease. CMC OA is partly mediated by joint contact stress, under which cell arrangement and metabolism are known to change. Whether mechanics at the joint level or biochemical composition at the microscopic level exhibit diverging patterns with sex, age, and pathology remains under continual investigation.

Since CMC OA is a degenerative disease of cartilage, the thickness of cartilage is a rudimentary indicator of health. Whether baseline cartilage thickness is different between men and women, whether there are changes with age, and whether there are changes with early stages of the disease are questions worth pursuing. In the current literature, there are few studies that have reported on the natural variation of CMC cartilage morphology among groups. Wear patterns in different stages of OA have been documented from excised trapezia and metacarpals [2, 3]. However, no studies have reported findings of sex-related or age-related morphological differences because CMC cartilage, with an average thickness of less than 1.0 mm [2, 3], is difficult to image and quantify accurately *in vivo* and because young cadaveric specimens with no signs of OA are challenging to acquire for *in vitro* analysis.

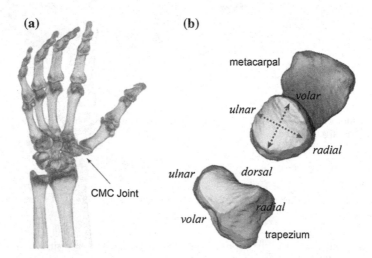

Fig. 1 **a** 3D rendering of the CT scan of a *right hand*, with the CMC joint highlighted and **b** an exploded view of the CMC joint with the subchondral mating surfaces highlighted

A feasible alternative to high resolution imaging of cartilage is to generate cartilage computationally by integrating multi-positional joint space volume information into one single cartilage model [4]. As part of an ongoing study on CMC joint kinematics we have collected sequential CT scans of the thumb of healthy subjects and patients with early signs of CMC OA in different positions. The purpose of the current study was to incorporate these data into subject-specific cartilage models and explore potential differences in the thickness of CMC cartilage, with sex, age, and early OA. We hypothesized that cartilage thickness would be lower in women than in men, lower in older than in younger subjects, and lower in patients with early OA than in normal subjects.

2 Methods

2.1 Subjects, Scanning, and Processing

22 asymptomatic subjects and 24 subjects with early OA—Eaton Stage I [5]—were recruited and examined by a board-certified orthopedic surgeon. The asymptomatic group included males and females from two age groups (younger—18 to 25 years—and older—45 to 75 years; Table 1).

After receiving IRB approval and informed consents, the thumb CMC joints in the dominant hands of asymptomatic subjects and the affected hands of OA patients were CT-scanned in 12 positions: a braced neutral position, four thumb range of motion positions (flexion, extension, abduction, adduction), and three functional task positions (jar grasp, key pinch, jar closing), with the last three in relaxed and loaded (80 % of their maximum load) conditions (Fig. 2). Image volumes were generated with a 16-slice clinical CT scanner (General Electric, Milwaukee, WI), at tube settings of 80 kVp and 40 mA, slice thickness of 0.625 mm, and in-plane resolution of 0.4 mm × 0.4 mm or better. The bones of the CMC joint—the trapezium and the first metacarpal—were segmented from the neutral scans using commercial software (Mimics®, Materialise, Leuven, Belgium) and 3-D bone models were exported as polygon meshes. Bone kinematics from the neutral position to all of the other positions were determined with a markerless bone registration algorithm [6]. The subchondral surfaces on the trapezium and first metacarpal were manually selected using Geomagic Studio® (Geomagic®, Research Triangle Park, NC) by carefully tracing the visible margins. Whole bone surface areas and subchondral surface areas were computed from the meshed surfaces.

Table 1 Mean age (±SD) of the subjects, grouped by sex (M: males, F: females), age group (Y: younger, O: older), and health group (N: normal, A: arthritic)

Sex		Age		Health	
M (11)	F (11)	Y (11)	O (11)	N (22)	A (24)
37.2 ± 14.2	38.7 ± 16.3	23.6 ± 1.5	52.4 ± 15.0	38.0 ± 14.2	54.3 ± 7.4

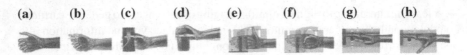

Fig. 2 3D rendering of the CT scans of one subject during **a** the neutral position, **b** key pinch, **c** jar grasp, **d** jar twist, **e** extension, **f** flexion, **g** adduction, **h** abduction

2.2 Cartilage Models

The cartilages on the trapezial and metacarpal articulating surfaces were modeled as meshless incompressible height fields, which were derived from joint space volume computations across the 12 scanned positions [4]. Briefly, the cartilage generation algorithm, which has been previously validated with *in vitro* μCT data and shown to have a mean accuracy of 0.02 mm, computes the minimum bone-to-bone distance at each vertex of the subchondral bone surface meshes, for each of the 12 positions. The minimum bone-to-bone distance of each vertex, across all the positions, is halved, and a height field assembled from all the points is used as an estimate of the computer-generated cartilage model on each mating bone. The average cartilage thickness was defined as the mean value of the cartilage height field. Each cartilage model was further divided into four quadrants in order to determine region-specific thicknesses. A coordinate system centered at the inflection point of the saddle-shaped subchondral bone surface and running through the two principal directions of curvature on the surface (Fig. 1b) was used to define the four quadrants.

2.3 Statistical Analysis

Three-way ANOVAs were used to determine the effects of sex, age, and pathology on the overall trapezial and metacarpal whole bone surface areas, subchondral surface areas, average cartilage thicknesses, and the quadrant-specific average cartilage thicknesses. Repeated measures ANOVAs (trapezium and metacarpal cartilage were analyzed separately) were used to determine if there were statistically significant differences among the average cartilage thicknesses of each quadrant in healthy subjects. Statistical significance was set at $p < 0.05$. Linear regression analyses were used to identify any potential scaling of the subchondral surface area and average cartilage thickness with bone size.

3 Results

The whole bone surface areas and subchondral surface areas of both the trapezium and the first metacarpal were significantly larger in males than in females, but did not differ with age and pathology (Tables 2 and 3). Overall, the subchondral surface

Table 2 Trapezial mean (SD) whole bone surface area (WA); subchondral surface area (SA), average cartilage thickness (T), and average thicknesses of the specific cartilage quadrants (T_1—ulnar-dorsal, T_2—radial-dorsal, T_3—radial-volar, T_4—ulnar-volar), divided by group; statistically significant group differences are bolded

	Sex		Age		Health	
	M (11)	F (11)	Y (11)	O (11)	N (22)	A (24)
WA (mm^2)	**1116.10**	**873.88**	920.75	1047.20	983.98	1037.03
	(181.73)	**(127.61)**	(144.06)	(223.80)	(194.74)	(191.64)
SA (mm^2)	**165.92**	**138.75**	143.6	158.53	151.10	156.14
	(36.68)	**(22.91)**	(19.46)	(41.12)	(32.30)	(34.61)
T (mm)	0.35 (0.10)	0.35 (0.10)	0.34 (0.09)	0.36 (0.12)	0.35 (0.10)	0.28 (0.14)
T_1 (mm)	0.49 (0.20)	0.52 (0.14)	0.50 (0.15)	0.51 (0.18)	0.51 (0.16)	0.47 (0.19)
T_2 (mm)	0.29 (0.17)	0.25 (0.12)	0.27 (0.15)	0.27 (0.10)	0.27 (0.13)	0.21 (0.16)
T_3 (mm)	0.30 (0.10)	0.30 (0.16)	0.29 (0.15)	0.31 (0.12)	0.30 (0.14)	0.23 (0.18)
T_4 (mm)	0.46 (0.12)	0.42 (0.20)	0.44 (0.16)	0.43 (0.18)	0.44 (0.16)	0.37 (0.18)

Table 3 Metacarpal mean (SD) whole bone surface area (WA), subchondral surface area (SA), average cartilage thickness (T), and average thicknesses of the specific cartilage quadrants (T_1—ulnar-dorsal, T_2—radial-dorsal, T_3—radial-volar, T_4—ulnar-volar), divided by group; statistically significant group differences are bolded

	Sex		Age		Health	
	M (11)	F (11)	Y (11)	O (11)	N (22)	A (24)
WA (mm^2)	**2362.80**	**1947.70**	2050.60	2222.10	2136.40	2100.10
	(306.54)	**(265.49)**	(253.99)	(418.85)	(349.23)	(334.38)
SA (mm^2)	**160.46**	**139.28**	139.28	158.53	148.90	151.59
	(38.34)	**(21.04)**	(24.01)	(35.70)	(31.28)	(37.69)
T (mm)	0.38 ± 0.13	0.33 ± 0.11	0.34 ± 0.10	0.37 ± 0.14	0.35 ± 0.12	0.30 ± 0.15
T_1 (mm)	0.58 (0.17)	0.51 (0.11)	0.53 (0.13)	0.55 (0.16)	0.55 (0.14)	0.58 (0.20)
T_2 (mm)	0.35 (0.13)	0.30 (0.13)	0.31 (0.13)	0.33 (0.13)	0.32 (0.13)	0.35 (0.20)
T_3 (mm)	0.22 (0.11)	0.21 (0.16)	0.19 (0.12)	0.25 (0.15)	0.22 (0.14)	0.16 (0.16)
T_4(mm)	0.43 (0.17)	0.40 (0.17)	0.41 (0.18)	0.41 (0.16)	**0.41 (0.17)**	**0.25 (0.19)**

area increased linearly with whole bone surface area (r = 0.77, p < 0.001 for the trapezium Fig. 3a, and r = 0.66, p < 0.001 for the metacarpal, not shown).

The average thickness of both the trapezial and the metacarpal cartilage models did not differ with sex, age, or early OA (Tables 2 and 3). The average cartilage thickness did not scale with bone size in both the trapezium (r < 0.001, p = 0.996, Fig. 3b.) and the metacarpal (r = 0.105, p = 0.487, not shown). Arthritic subjects, however, had a higher variation in average cartilage thickness. The quadrant-specific average thickness also did not differ with sex and age in both of the cartilage models (Tables 2 and 3). On the metacarpal, however, the ulnar-volar quadrant was 39 % thinner in the arthritic subjects than in the normal subjects (Table 3; Fig. 4).

In the normal trapezial cartilage there was a significant difference between the average thicknesses of the ulnar quadrants and the radial quadrants (Table 2; Fig. 5).

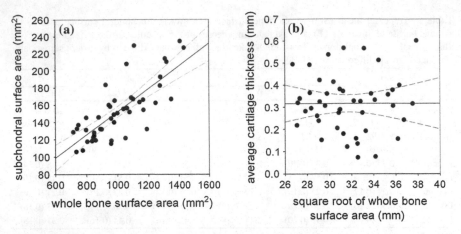

Fig. 3 **a** Trapezial subchondral surface area was strongly correlated with whole bone surface area; **b** cartilage thickness was not correlated with whole bone surface area (the square root of)

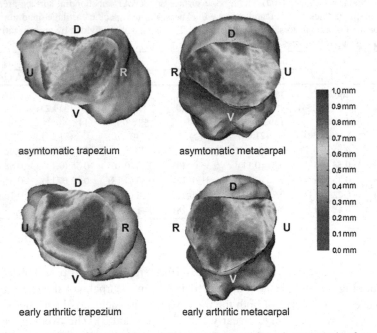

Fig. 4 The computationally generated cartilages on the trapezia and metacarpals of an asymptomatic subject and a patient with early OA, colored by thickness

In the metacarpal cartilage, however, there were significant differences among the thicknesses of all of the quadrants, with the thickness of the ulnar-dorsal quadrant being the highest, followed by that of the ulnar-volar, radial-dorsal, and radial-volar quadrants, in descending order (Table 3; Fig. 5).

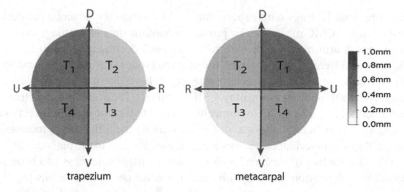

Fig. 5 A schematic representation of the average trapezial and metacarpal cartilage thickness of each of the four quadrants in healthy subjects: on the trapezium, both the radial quadrants were significantly thinner than the ulnar quadrants; on the metacarpal the ulnar-dorsal quadrant was the thickest, followed by the ulnar-volar, radial-dorsal, and radial-volar, in descending order

4 Discussion

The thumb CMC joint is the most common site of reconstructive surgery in the upper extremity due to the pain and loss of thumb function associated with CMC osteoarthritis [7]. Understanding cartilage wear patters with OA progression and morphological baseline differences in populations that are more predisposed to OA would provide valuable insight into the mechanics of the disease. Since CMC cartilage is difficult to image and quantify *in vivo*, the purpose of this study was to use a subject-specific model, which has been previously validated, to gain insight onto the morphology of thumb CMC cartilage. Using CT data from 12 physiological positions, in a cohort of 46 subjects, we set to determine if there were any sex-, age-, or early OA-related differences in CMC cartilage thickness. We found no sex- or age-related differences, but found that the ulnar-volar quadrant of the metacarpal cartilage of patients with early OA was significantly thinner than its counterpart in asymptomatic subjects. We also found that in asymptomatic individuals the ulnar-dorsal quadrants had the highest thickness and the radial-volar quadrants had the lowest, in both the trapezial and metacarpal cartilages.

Our findings of thickness patterns were generally consistent with findings from previous cadaveric studies on CMC cartilage wear with different stages of OA [2, 3]. While no previous studies have compared the cartilage thickness of normal subjects with that of arthritic subjects, studies of cartilage in cadaveric specimens with different stages of OA have concluded that cartilage is thinnest in the radial-volar quadrant with Stage I OA and that wear progresses onto the ulnar-volar quadrant, starting with the metacarpal first [2]. It is therefore reasonable that both healthy and early arthritic subjects have thinner cartilage in the radial-volar quadrant, but that with OA, the cartilage in the volar-ulnar quadrant of the metacarpal is thinner than in asymptomatic subjects. These findings are important because they complement previous findings with *in vivo* data and because they advance the current understanding of CMC mechanics by providing baseline data on cartilage thickness variation in non-arthritic subjects, which had not been documented before.

The lack of differences between the sex and age groups was intriguing and while it may be due to an insufficient sample size, we believe that it is representative of the underlying morphology of healthy CMC cartilage. These findings advance the general understanding of CMC joint mechanics and OA pathogenesis by verifying that metabolic, genetic, or hormonal differences, under the influence of mechanical loading, rather than mechanical factors alone, are implicated in the pathoetiology of CMC OA. Our finding of no correlation between cartilage thickness and bone size is consistent with previous studies with similar conclusions in other joints [8].

A few limitations must be considered when interpreting our findings. First, as mentioned above, it may be possible that there are sex- or age-related differences that may have not been captured with our sample size. Further studies with more subjects may be required for more conclusive results. Second, the cartilage computation algorithm depends on the scanned positions. This algorithm operates under the assumption that through a wide range of position, the greater part of the articular surfaces must come into contact, therefore more positions would increase the robustness of the cartilage thickness estimation. We believe that the set of the 12 chosen positions was diverse and included extreme range of motion positions (flexion, extension, abduction, adduction), which likely placed most of the mating articular surfaces into contact.

Ongoing work includes expanding the sample size and tracking the arthritic patients at 1.5 and 3 years from the baseline time point. *In vivo* longitudinal data on cartilage thickness and wear with OA progression would answer important questions on the pathomechanics of CMC OA. Findings from these studies have the potential to influence CMC OA management in non-end stage cases, whereas the cartilage model applied here can be further incorporated into subject-specific simulations of thumb mechanics and offers the opportunity of developing statistical models of CMC cartilage for usage in clinical OA staging, if combined with dynamic volume CT.

Acknowledgments This work was supported by NIH AR059185. The authors would like to thank A. Garcia, J.B. Schwartz, J.C. Tarrant, B.J. Wilcox, Drs. A-P.C. Weiss, A.L. Ladd, C.J. Got, and E.G. Marai for their contributions to this work.

References

1. Haara MM, Heliövaara M, Kröger H, Arokoski JPA, Manninen P, Kärkkäinen A, Knekt P, Impivaara O, Aromaa A (2004) Osteoarthritis in the carpometacarpal joint of the thumb. Prevalence and associations with disability and mortality. J Bone Joint Surg Am 86-A:1452–1457
2. Koff MF, Ugwonali OF, Strauch RJ, Rosenwasser MP, Ateshian GA, Mow VC (2003) Sequential wear patterns of the articular cartilage of the thumb carpometacarpal joint in osteoarthritis. J Hand Surg Am 28:597–604
3. Ateshian GA, Ark JW, Rosenwasser MP, Pawluk RJ, Soslowsky LJ, Mow VC (1995) Contact areas in the thumb carpometacarpal joint. J Orthop Res 13:450–458

4. Marai GE, Crisco JJ, Laidlaw DH (2006) A kinematics-based method for generating cartilage maps and deformations in the multi-articulating wrist joint from CT images. Conf Proc IEEE Eng Med Biol Soc 1:2079–2082
5. Eaton RG, Glickel SZ (1987) Trapeziometacarpal osteoarthritis. Staging as a rationale for treatment. Hand Clin 3:455–471
6. Marai GE, Laidlaw DH, Crisco JJ (2006) Super-resolution registration using tissue-classified distance fields. IEEE Trans Med Imaging 25:177–187
7. Acheson RM, Chan YK, Clemett AR (1970) New Haven survey of joint diseases. XII. Distribution and symptoms of osteoarthrosis in the hands with reference to handedness. Ann Rheum Dis 29:275–286
8. Faber SC, Eckstein F, Lukasz S, Mühlbauer R, Hohe J, Englmeier K-H, Reiser M (2001) Gender differences in knee joint cartilage thickness, volume and articular surface areas: assessment with quantitative three-dimensional MR imaging. Skeletal Radiol 30:144–150

Patient Specific Modeling of Pectus Excavatum for the Nuss Procedure Simulation

Krzysztof J. Rechowicz, Mohammad F. Obeid and Frederic D. McKenzie

Abstract Patient specific models are crucial for both simulation and surgical planning. It is not different for the Nuss procedure, which is a minimally invasive surgery for correcting pectus excavatum (PE)—a congenital chest wall deformity. Typically, patients differ not only in size but also severity of the chest depression and type of the deformity, making the simulation process challenging. In this paper, we approach the problem of a patient specific model creation resulting in the development of a parameterized model of the human torso including the ribcage. All the parameters are obtainable from pre-surgical CT. In order to validate our model, we compared the simulated shape of the chest with surface scans obtained from PE patients for both pre- and post-surgery. Results showed that both shapes are in agreement in the area of the deformity, making this method valid for the need of simulating the Nuss procedure.

1 Introduction

No surgery is risk free. Even fairly simple procedures can have a significant death rate and other serious complications may arise. However, these risks can be minimized by developing appropriate surgical planning and simulation. One of the key steps in the development of a simulation is providing a patient specific model including appropriate pathologies.

K. J. Rechowicz (✉) · M. F. Obeid · F. D. McKenzie
Department of Modeling, Simulation, and Visualization Engineering,
Old Dominion University, Norfolk, VA 23508, USA
e-mail: krechowi@odu.edu

M. F. Obeid
e-mail: mobei001@odu.edu

F. D. McKenzie
rdmckenz@odu.edu

J. M. R. S. Tavares et al. (eds.), *Bio-Imaging and Visualization for Patient-Customized Simulations*, Lecture Notes in Computational Vision and Biomechanics 13, DOI: 10.1007/978-3-319-03590-1_10, © Springer International Publishing Switzerland 2014

We seek this risk mitigation strategy for the minimally invasive technique for the repair of pectus excavatum (MIRPE), often referred to as the Nuss procedure. Pectus excavatum (PE), also called sunken or funnel chest, is a congenital chest wall deformity which is characterized, in most cases, by a deep depression of the sternum. This condition affects primarily children and young adults and is responsible for about 90 % of congenital chest wall abnormalities [4]. Typically, this deformity can be found in approximately one in every 400 births and is inherited in many instances [5]. Very often other problems can accompany this condition, like scoliosis and breathing issues.

Cartoski et al. classified PE using the following criteria: localized versus diffuse depression, also known as cup versus saucer, length of the depression, symmetry, sternal torsion, slope and position of absolute depth, and unique patterns of the deformation [2]. Frequency distribution of subtypes of typical PE and rare types was recently performed by Kelly et al. on a random sample of 300 patients with nonsyndromic PE [3]. Over two-thirds of patients were characterized by the cup type PE, whereas 21 % by the saucer type PE. The remaining 11 % were characterized by the trench type PE and very rare Currarino-Silverman which is a mix between PE and pectus carinatum (PC). The deepest point of PE was in the majority of cases shifted to the right of the midline, whereas, shifted to left and central represented equally 20 %. Almost in all cases, the deepest point was in the lower part of the sternum.

Among various PE treatments options, the Nuss procedure, has been proven to have a high success rate, satisfactory aesthetic outcome and low interference with skeletal growth as specified in [5]. The Nuss procedure starts with small bilateral incisions on the side of the torso aligning with the deepest point of the depression. Using a surgical tool, the surgeon opens a pathway from the incision, down between the ribs, under the sternum, taking care not to puncture the lungs or heart, back up through the ribs and out the opposite incision. Then, a steel bar, previously bent to suit the patient, is pulled through the pathway. At this time, if the position of the bar is correct, the surgeon can slowly elevate the bar to loosen the cartilage connections within the inner thorax. After this step, the concave bar is then flipped convex, so that the arch elevates and supports the sternum in a normal position. The bar is then sutured into place, often with the addition of a stabilizer to prevent movement. In some cases when PE is severe or when a patient is adult, a second and even a third bar may be inserted. After a period of at least 2 years, the bar is removed, resulting in a largely permanent result. Rechowicz et al. showed the need for simulating the Nuss procedure and outlined a design and validation methodology of such simulator that, to our knowledge, has not been fulfilled to date [6]. A hardware setup was built to implement the Nuss procedure simulator, including two displays for external and internal view, a high-force haptic device to enable force-feedback, and inertial tracker to simulate the thoracoscope (Fig. 1). One of the key components of successful simulation is the ability to reproduce a variety of patient specific models in a simple way which also has not been pursued so far. In this paper, we focus on the development of a patient specific model for the need of simulating the Nuss procedure and we will present comparisons between the simulated chest shapes and patients surface scans.

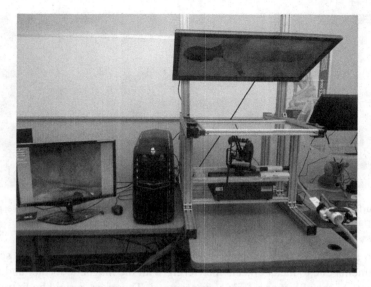

Fig. 1 Hardware setup for the Nuss procedure simulator

2 Methodology

The methods used to construct models of PE are now introduced as well as the approaches and techniques undertaken to develop patient-specific simulated chest shapes for the Nuss procedure. First presented is the collection and processing of patient information in the form of CT and surface scans. The development of the generic model of the ribcage and torso is then described as well as the extraction of corresponding patient-specific parameters and metrics. Lastly, the design of a comparison and evaluation platform is introduced where the actual and simulated models are compared and assessed.

2.1 Data Acquisition and Processing

From 2007, we have been collecting surface scans, using a FastScan laser scanner (Polhemus, VT, USA), from patients with PE before and after the Nuss procedure (EVMS IRB# 07-08-EX-0202). Pre-surgical scans were obtained just prior to the surgery, whereas post-surgical surface scan was performed either 6 months after the surgery during routine check up or just before the bar removal surgery approximately 2 years after bar placement. Included within each scan are three markers related to features on the surface of the chest, i.e. the nipples and the navel, which allows to register pre- and post-surgical scans and identify a growth factor in between each scanning.

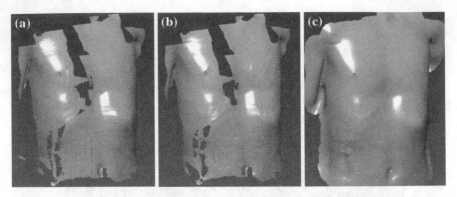

Fig. 2 Surface scan: **a** raw scan with registered sweeps, **b** surface built from merged sweeps, and **c** RBF surface approximation

When a handheld 3D scanner is used, existence of small errors in the scanner measurements due to metal objects interfering with the magnetic locater and minor movements of the object or reference is assumed. Therefore, a rigid body transformation is applied to each sweep that a scan is consisted of (Fig. 2a). The surface model of skin is built next directly from a point cloud represented by sweeps, which are merged (Fig. 2b). Smoothing factor has to be controlled in this process so that the surface is regular enough, even when sweeps are not aligned perfectly. A surface created by simple joining points belonging to a cloud may still contain holes and defects, which would require significant amount of work. Therefore, we utilized a fast RBF interpolation technique, incorporated into scanning software, to fill holes and smooth scans if necessary (Fig. 2c). Optionally, if smoothing applied by the RBF interpolation technique is too high, an alternative way to fill holes in models similar to chest scans can be used [7].

Additionally, for each patient, we obtained a pre-surgical CT and post-surgical X-ray. The pre-surgical CT is typically performed 6 months prior to the surgery, whereas x-rays are taken within 2 days after the surgery. It would be beneficial to obtain post-surgical CT but it is not routinely performed due to cost and exposure to additional radiation.

Each subject's deformity has been previously classified in the picture archiving and communication system (PACS) by cup, saucer or unknown, and symmetric or asymmetric criteria. For the purpose of this study, we chose patients characterized by the symmetric deformity type, which resulted in four patients with saucer and two with cup type deformity.

2.2 Generic Model of the Ribcage and Torso

In order to overcome the problem of missing elements corresponding to the cartilage when the ribcage is segmented from CT data and to provide a regular geometry of the ribcage model, we used a female skeletal model created based on Visible Human

Project [1]. For the torso, we used a generic low polygon model which was adjusted to a skinny posture in horizontal position.

An underlying system of bones was constructed. A bones system is a jointed set of objects called bones which is typically used to animate various objects, especially those described by a continuous mesh. The translation and rotation of bones is typically performed using forward and inverse kinematics. Before the model can be deformed using bones, envelopes associated with each bone have to be defined. The envelope is the tool for controlling deformation of the surface of a model, called in this process skin. An envelope defines an area of influence of a single bone. Vertices bounded by the envelopes are assigned weights to generate smooth transitions at the joints. The envelopes and weights were defined based on characteristics of both types of deformations presented introduced by [2] and CT data collected for this study. This process is very tedious but vitally important as it is responsible for the generation of realistic deformations.

As can be seen in Fig. 3, vertices within an outer envelope do not receive 100 % weighting. Weights fall off sigmoidally for the saucer in the area between the inner and outer envelope boundaries (Fig. 3a, b) and fast out for cups (Fig. 3c, d).

2.3 Parameters for the Patient Specific Model

In order to create a patient specific model, the shape of the ribcage and torso is controlled by non-uniform scaling in the x, y and z-axes. Width and depth of the ribcage is measured on a CT slice approximately at the point of the highest depression, i.e. where the sternum reaches the highest distance from the normal position (Fig. 4a). From the same slice where the width and depth are measured, sternum displacement and torsion is obtained as shown in Fig. 4b. Height of the ribcage is based on the length of the sternum. This is calculated by registering the CT slices where the beginning and the end of the sternum can be observed. Knowing the distance between slices, the overall length of the sternum can be then calculated. Classification between a barrel and oval ribcage directly depends on the ratio between width and depth. As that ratio increases, a ribcage tends to follow an oval shape.

In order to define patient specific PE deformation, it is essential to specify parameters for measurement that can be quantified and used to accurately reproduce the deformity. One parameter is depression, which is a measure of the distance between the ribs-line and the position of the sunken sternum taken from the CT layer where the rest of the parameters are measured (Fig. 4). For the depression parameter, simply measuring the deepest point of the sternum in the CT image will produce an error. This error can be analyzed when considering a sagittal view of the sternum (Fig. 5).

We define the axis of a normal sternum to be the line AB and the axis of a deformed sternum to be the line AC both of length a. Connecting the two lines with line BC results in an isosceles triangle $\triangle ABC$. $\angle CAB$ is the angle of sternum depression which is the measure that we need as the bone and envelop for the ribcage model can be deformed by rotation. We will call this angle α.

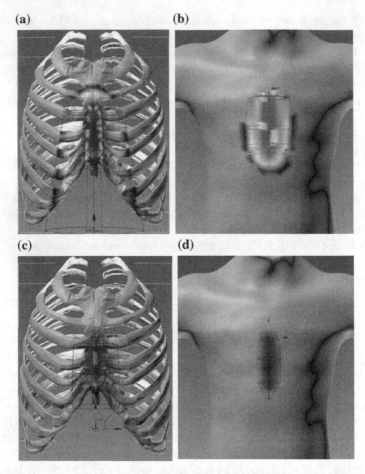

Fig. 3 Envelopes for: **a** saucer type PE ribcage, **b** saucer type PE torso, **c** cup type PE ribcage, and **d** cup type PE torso

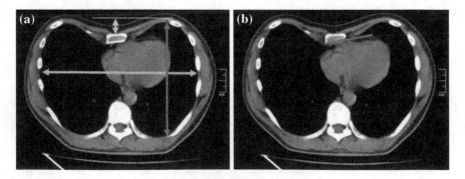

Fig. 4 CT measurements: **a** width, depth, depression, **b** sternal torsion

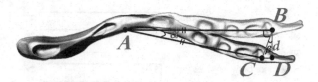

Fig. 5 Depression calculation parameters

The CT image, however, only provides a transverse view which means that when a linear measurement is made, it gives the length of line BD which we will define as the linear distance of depression d. A mathematical operation is needed to convert this linear distance to an angle. In addition, merely using this calculated angle for depression assumes that the depression results in a vertical drop of point B which means that, since the sides AB and AC are of equal and fixed length, points C and D are in the same point in space. This is not true. Another step will therefore follow to compensate for that difference.

First the value of angle α is to be estimated given the linear distance of depression d. To do so, the isosceles triangle $\triangle ABC$ is considered. In order to find the value of α, we assume temporarily that BC is equal to BD. The error produced by this assumption will be compensated for in the following step. Using the Law of Cosines, we can come to

$$d^2 = AB^2 + AC^2 - 2 * AB * AC * \cos \alpha, \tag{1}$$

which gives

$$\alpha = \cos^{-1}\left(1 - \frac{d^2}{2a^2}\right). \tag{2}$$

After knowing the value of the angle α, this information can be used to calculate the actual length of the side BC, which we will call $\hat{d}$, by considering both $\triangle ABC$ and $\triangle BCD$. From $\triangle ABC$ we can see

$$\angle ABC + \angle ACB + \alpha = 180°, \tag{3}$$

Since $\angle ABC = \angle ACB$,

$$\angle ABC = \frac{180° - \alpha}{2}. \tag{4}$$

Therefore,

$$\beta = \frac{\alpha}{2}. \tag{5}$$

Using this result in $\triangle BCD$,

$$\cos \beta = \frac{d}{\hat{d}}, \tag{6}$$

which gives

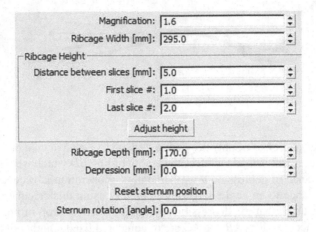

Fig. 6 Patient specific parameters input window

$$\hat{d} = \frac{d}{\cos \beta}. \tag{7}$$

We then use the new value $\hat{d}$ to calculate the depression angle α. This value of the angle will be used as the depression parameter.

Another parameter for deformation is the sternum torsion which can be simply measured from the CT slice used as it shows the amount of torsion that the sternum undergoes. Thus, the patient specific information collected in the previous steps are shape parameters including width, length and depth as well as deformation parameters including depression and torsion. To deploy these values to the patient's avatar in the simulation, the environment had to be constructed to receive them as input parameters. Applying the shape parameters is trivial as they can be computed as scaling factors for the model in the x, y and z dimension. For the deformation parameters, a script was developed that would allow the user to enter the value of depression, which is internally converted to α, as well as the value for the sternal torsion (Fig. 6). This script directly affects the bone and envelope system to make the model automatically conform to the patient specific information collected.

2.4 Evaluation of the Patient Specific Model

To evaluate a patient specific model, we compared it with the pre-surgical scan for the same patient and presented it in a form of a colormap. This resulted in four patients with saucer type deformity and two patients with cup type deformity and presented it in a form of a color map. Additionally, we recorded the difference between simulated shape of the chest and the actual result of the surgery at the point corresponding to the CT slice where the initial parameters were measured.

For each patient, we created a colormap projected onto their post-surgical surface scan which was scaled to their pre-surgical scan to compensate for patient growth thus objectively measuring the post-surgical improvement. Additionally, for those patients we compared pre- and post-surgical scans to calculate the displacement that occurred from the point corresponding to the cross-section where the pre-surgical parameters were taken. Since that point moves the same distance as the internal point on the sternum, we were able to observe decrease in depression after the Nuss procedure. Eventually, we compared simulated chest shape with the post-surgical shape and recorded the difference as in the case for the pre-surgical shape.

3 Results and Discussion

After developing a mechanism for generating patient-specific models and patient-customized pre- and post-surgical PE deformations, the corresponding results for the subjects of this study are evaluated and compared for validity. For each subject, pre-surgical results of the simulated models will be compared with pre-surgical surface scans and the same for post-surgical results.

3.1 Pre-surgical Patient Specific Model

In order to evaluate the ability of our generic model to conform to patient's size and deformation, we compared generated deformity with the actual shape of the chest in the form of a surface scan. Figure 7 shows results of such comparisons for the saucer and cup type PE. In the case of the saucer type, it can be seen that the overall difference between simulated shape of the chest is close to 0 (Fig. 7b) which is the most important indicator from the clinical point of view. The slight difference in the lower rib region can be caused by the characteristics of the scanning procedure where a subject lays down with arms by his torso and a slight inspiration. Our model is adjusted to the characteristics of the Nuss procedure where the arms are spread almost 90 degrees with respect to the torso. In the case of the cup type PE, the difference along the centerline is slightly higher and equal to approximately 4 mm. However, the deformity itself is characterized by differences close to 0 (Fig. 7d).

To better evaluate our results, we recorded in Table 1 the difference between both surfaces at the point corresponding to the CT slice where the measurements were taken. Subjects 1–5 represent saucer type PE, whereas subjects 6 and 7 represent cup type PE. The highest negative difference, 4.2 mm, was observed for subject 3. However, it is very localized and does not significantly affect the overall difference between both shapes which is close to 0.

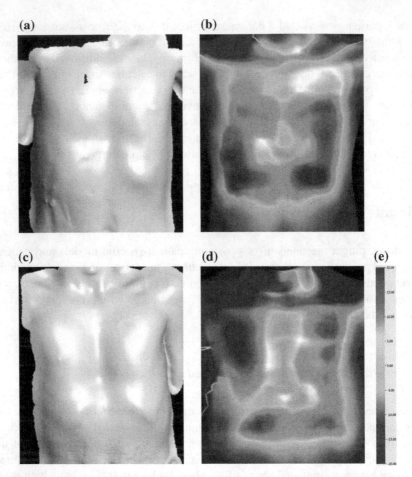

Fig. 7 Pre-surgical: **a** saucer type PE surface scan, **b** comparison between simulated and actual chest shape (**a**), **c** cup type PE surface scan, **d** comparison between simulated and actual chest shape (**c**), and **e** scale in mm

Table 1 Comparison results

Subject	Pre-surgical simulated chest shape versus surface scan (mm)	Post-surgical simulated chest shape versus surface scan (mm)	Pre- versus post-surgical surface scan (mm)
1	1.72	5.8	46
2	3.2	−3.2	36
3	−3.8	−1	37
4	1.8	−5	32
5	4.2	−3.2	26
6	3.2	3	40

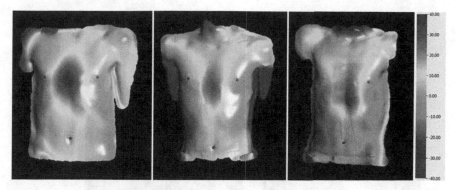

Fig. 8 Pre- and post-surgical surface scan comparison, scale in mm

3.2 Pre- and Post-surgical Scan Comparison

Pre- and post-surgical scans were compared to calculate the sternum position after the surgery. Figure 8 shows such comparisons for a sample of subjects. The results are in agreement with the characteristics of the Nuss procedure where the most dramatic change in chest shape was in the area of PE. The difference between pre- and post-surgical chest shape at the point corresponding to the CT slice where the initial parameters were measured are presented in Table 1. This change was also confirmed by measurements taken form the post-surgical latero-lateral X-rays. This information was used to determine the position of the sternum for each patient after correction.

3.3 Post-surgical Patient Specific Model

As far as the post-surgical patient specific model is concerned, Fig. 9b shows good approximation of the actual post-surgical chest shape in the area for saucer type PE by the patient specific model. The difference in the lower part of the ribcage has the same source as for the pre-surgical comparison, i.e. horizontal position of a patient and slight inspiration differences. The higher difference around the point below the xyphoid process position is caused by the presence of the ridge in the actual chest shape, whereas in the patient specific model this region is not affected by the sternum movement. Since this point is below the deformity, it is not crucial for the simulation.

Figure 9d shows the comparison for the post-surgical cup type PE. Both shapes are in agreement in the area of the deformity and ribs. A higher difference is visible in the area of the lower torso below the line of ribs. This difference comes from the inspiration of the patient as visible in Fig. 9c and is not relevant to the Nuss procedure itself. The maximum difference between both shapes at the point corresponding to the CT slice where the initial measurements were taken is shown in Table 1. For all

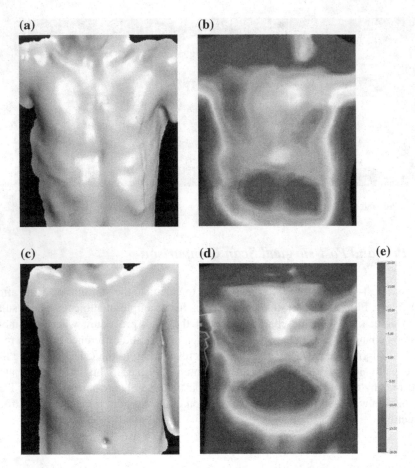

Fig. 9 Post-surgical: **a** saucer type PE surface scan, **b** comparison between simulated and actual chest shape (**a**), **c** cup type PE surface scan, **d** comparison between simulated and actual chest shape (**c**), and **e** scale in mm

subjects, the maximum difference is very localized and situated in the same area which is not very significant when the surgical outcome is evaluated. Overall, the difference between both chest shapes is close to 0($<$0.5 mm).

4 Conclusions

In this paper, we presented a methodology for the development of a patient specific model corresponding to a person with PE that is needed for both surgical simulation and planning. We proposed a parameterized system to create a patient specific ribcage, torso, and PE deformity. We compared our results with the actual torso shapes in a form of a surface scan. Using a colormap to evaluate the difference between the simulated and actual shape of the chest, we were able to show good approximation of our model for both saucer and cup type PE. Additionally, based on information from the comparison between pre- and post-surgical surface scan, we simulated the post-surgical shape of the chest and compared it with the actual outcomes of the surgery. The overall difference between both shapes was in the range of 3–4 showing good prognosis for the use in the simulation of the Nuss procedure. Collecting more pre- and post-surgical surface scans from more subjects in the future will enhance comprehensiveness of the experiment.

References

1. Ackerman M (1998) The visible human project. Proc IEEE 86(3):504–511. doi:10.1109/5. 662875
2. Cartoski MJ, Nuss D, Goretsky MJ, Proud VK, Croitoru DP, Gustin T, Mitchell K, Vasser E, Kelly RE (2006) Classification of the dysmorphology of pectus excavatum. J Pediatr Surg 41(9):1573–1581. doi:10.1016/j.jpedsurg.2006.05.055. http://dx.doi.org/10.1016/j.jpedsurg.2006.05.055
3. Kelly RE, Quinn A, Varela P, Redlinger RE, Nuss D (2013) Dysmorphology of chest wall deformities: frequency distribution of subtypes of typical pectus excavatum and rare subtypes. Arch Bronconeumol (English Version) 49(05):196–200
4. Pretorius ES, Haller JA, Fishman EK (1998) Spiral ct with 3d reconstruction in children requiring reoperation for failure of chest wall growth after pectus excavatum surgery. Preliminary observations. Clin Imaging 22(2):108–116
5. Protopapas AD, Athanasiou T (2008) Peri-operative data on the nuss procedure in children with pectus excavatum: independent survey of the first 20 years' data. J Cardiothorac Surg 3:40. doi:10.1186/1749-8090-3-40. http://dx.doi.org/10.1186/1749-8090-3-40
6. Rechowicz K, McKenzie F (2011) A strategy for simulating and validating the nuss procedure for the minimally invasive correction of pectus excavatum. In: 2011 4th international conference on biomedical engineering and informatics (BMEI) vol. 4, pp 2370–2374 doi:10.1109/BMEI. 2011.6098771
7. Rechowicz KJ, Kelly R, Goretsky M, Frantz FW, Knisley S, Nuss D, McKenzie FD (2010) Development of an average chest shape for objective evaluation of the aesthetic outcome in the nuss procedure planning process. In: Proceedings of southern biomedical, engineering conference 2010

Formulating a Pedicle Screw Fastening Strength Surrogate via Patient-Specific Virtual Templating and Planning

Cristian A. Linte, Jon J. Camp, Kurt Augustine, Paul M. Huddleston, Anthony A. Stans, David R. Holmes III and Richard A. Robb

Abstract Traditional 2D images provide limited use for accurate planning of spine interventions, mainly due to the complex 3D anatomy of the and spine, and close proximity of nerve bundles and vascular structures that must be avoided during the procedure. Our clinician-friendly platform for spine surgery planning takes advantage of 3D pre-operative images, to enable oblique reformatting and 3D rendering of individual or multiple vertebrae, interactive templating and placement of virtual pedicle implants, and provide surrogate estimates of the "fastening strength" of implanted pedicle screws based on implant dimension and bone mineral density of the displaced bone substrate. Preliminary studies using retrospective clinical data have demonstrated the feasibility of the platform in assisting the surgeon with selection of appropriate size implant and trajectory that provides optimal "fastening strength", given the intrinsic vertebral geometry and bone mineral density.

1 Introduction

Spinal deformity correction procedures via pedicle screws and rods have traditionally been planned using 2D radiographs, an approach which has proved inadequate for precise planning due to the complex 3D anatomy of the vertebrae, the spinal column itself, and the close proximity of the nerve bundles, blood vessels and viscera, that must be avoided during surgery [1–5]. Hence, penetration of the anterior cortex of the vertebral bodies could also lead to injury of one or more of these vessels. As such,

C. A. Linte (✉) · J. J. Camp · K. Augustine · D. R. Holmes III · R. A. Robb
Biomedical Imaging Resource, Mayo Clinic, Rochester, MN, USA
e-mail: linte.cristian@mayo.edu

D. R. Holmes III
e-mail: holmes.david3@mayo.edu

P. M. Huddleston · Anthony A. Stans
Division of Orthopedic Surgery, Mayo Clinic, Rochester, MN, USA

J. M. R. S. Tavares et al. (eds.), *Bio-Imaging and Visualization for Patient-Customized Simulations*, Lecture Notes in Computational Vision and Biomechanics 13, DOI: 10.1007/978-3-319-03590-1_11, © Springer International Publishing Switzerland 2014

significant care must be taken to avoid the risk of neural or vascular damage during intervention.

Considering these limitations, it is critical for the surgeon to have access to superior images of the patient-specific anatomy that display the 3D relationships between these structures and enable intuitive, efficient and risk-free planning. As part of current clinical practice, 3D imaging scans, such as computed tomography (CT) and magnetic resonance imaging (MRI), are typically acquired prior to spine correction procedures to help plan the intervention. During the planning process, which usually takes place in the operating room (OR) just prior to the procedure, the axial images are reviewed and critical vertebrae are identified. To select the appropriate pedicle screw size (diameter and length), the depth of the vertebra (i.e., distance from pedicles to anterior surface of the vertebral body) is measured, as well as the width of the pedicle at its narrowest point. The angle of approach is determined by an estimated deviation from the spinous process. Consistent with current clinical practice based on the review of the 2D axial slices of the anatomy, the dimensions of the proposed screws, along with the insertion angles, are documented by hand on a planning form. Nevertheless, due to the intrinsic curvature of the spine, vertebral axis and body axis do not usually coincide and therefore axial CT image slices cannot provide true measurements of the vertebral body or pedicle, which may in turn lead to inadequate decisions with regards to pedicle screw size and trajectory.

In response to these challenges and driven by the motivation and insight of our orthopedic surgery collaborators, we have developed and published on a clinical application that provides full 3D visualization for superior surgical planning. The platform uses routine 3D CT data to generate detailed virtual plans of the instrumentation procedures, enabling the identification of the appropriate size implant and angle of approach, based on the geometry of the vertebra. In this paper, we extend the existing platform to include a surrogate measure of the achieved "fastening strength" as a means to provide additional feedback with regards to screw placement.

While we recognize ongoing efforts in computer-assisted spine surgery to assist the surgeon with actual implant positioning during the procedure, we believe that such endeavours, although valuable, make no direct attempt to improve procedure planning and eventually "remove" the planning process out of the OR and reduce time-to-incision, anaesthesia time, and overall procedure time and costs. Although 2D templating methods for orthopedic implants has been utilized for quite some time, our proposed application integrates new and advanced visualization and planning that entails 3D virtual modeling and templating capabilities. In its current form, this tool allows surgeons to plan an intervention *pre-operatively*, outside of the OR, using objective measures to identify the optimal size and trajectory for safe and secure implant positioning.

Herein we describe the platform infrastructure and capabilities, present preliminary studies based on retrospective clinical data designed to assess the platform performance relative to standard clinical outcome of typical instrumentation procedures, and share our initial clinical experience in employing this platform to plan several complicated spinal correction procedures for which the traditional planning approaches proved insufficient.

2 Methodology

2.1 Spine Surgery Planning Platform

Most advanced tools lack widespread clinical acceptance, as physicians have limited time to become familiar with new and complicated software applications. Our goal is to provide a powerful tool that addresses the clinical challenges, fits seamlessly into the typical procedure workflow, and is intuitive and simple to use. The application is developed within a comprehensive, mature clinical imaging toolkit [6] designed to provide powerful image visualization and analysis tools as part of an intuitive and easy-to-use interface [7]. Its underlying architecture is based on a concept familiar to physicians, where each case is associated with a specific patient and clinical workflow.

2.2 Procedure Planning

The platform runs on a standard desktop computer; patient CT or MR image data can be imported directly from an institutional PACS server. The planning process is conducted in a two steps for each vertebra. In the first step, each vertebra is reoriented such that the axial image plane is perpendicular to its central axis. The user identifies a bounding box based on the sagittal and coronal views, and aligns its edges with the vertebral end-plates to ensure full enclosure of the vertebral body, as well as any part of the implant that may extend outside the vertebra, such as pedicle screw heads. The reorientation is rapidly performed via a simple GUI that requires 2–3 mouse clicks in each of the two views. Following realignment, the *true* pedicle length and width at its narrowest point (i.e., screw length and diameter) are determined, along with the angle of approach (i.e., screw trajectory).

In the second step, digital templates of pedicle screws are selected from a virtual pedicle screw template library that contains several standard instrumentation products, including different vendor and screw geometries. A pedicle screw type of desired size is selected and virtually "inserted" into the axial image. Optimal placement within the vertebra is achieved by interactively translating or rotating the implant in any of the three orthogonal views, as demonstrated in Fig. 1, while panning through the dataset for visual verification throughout the entire extent of the pedicle screw. Exact dimensions and angles of approach for each implanted screw are automatically determined upon final positioning and recorded in the planning report—the planning "recipe"—generated by the spine surgery planning tool. The report provides a list of all instrumented vertebral segments, templated screw type and manufacturer, screw dimensions (i.e., diameter and length), and the insertion trajectory defined by the axial and sagittal angles measured relative to the vertebral axis. In addition to the implant list, the report also contains a collection of bi-planar images showing each instrumented vertebral segment.

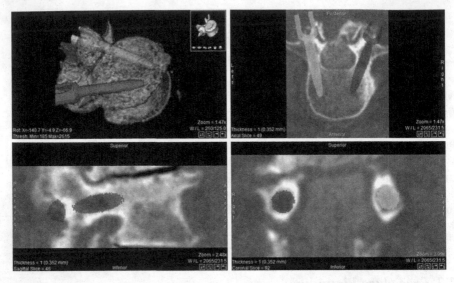

Fig. 1 Virtual screw templates are placed interactively into the image data. Each template corresponds to a particular implant manufacturer. The virtual implant is evaluated in both the orthogonal 2D image slices and 3D renderings to ensure correct length and width

2.3 Virtual Templating and 3D Subject-Specific Modeling

The final step of the pre-operative plan is to produce a digital volume-rendered patient-specific 3D model of the spine along with the virtual models of the inserted pedicle screws (Fig. 2), which can be used along with the generated report to prepare the instrumentation inventory for the operation [8–10]. Not only is such level of detail not available using traditional 2D planning methods, but the digital plan can also be easily translated [8–10] into a full-size physical patient-specific model of the virtually instrumented spine using 3D printing or rapid prototyping. The physical model can be used to better understand the anatomy, practice prior to the intervention, or assist the surgical team in the OR with real-time visualization and guidance for implant placement.

2.4 Estimation of Fastening Strength

According to strength of materials principles and theories of failure, each screw withstands a maximum force before it can be torn away from the threaded holes that were created in the material during its insertion. The holding power of a typical screw depends on the dimensions of the screw, the insertion depth, and the material properties (typically characterized by specific gravity) of the the material in which it is inserted. By transposing this theory to the pedicle screw implantation scenario, its holding power is directly proportional to the screw diameter (D), the bone-inserted screw length (L), as well as the specific gravity (i.e., bone mineral density) of the

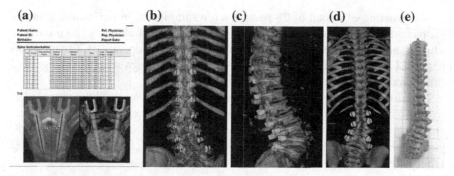

Fig. 2 **a** Example of automatically generated report including a complete list of all implants and labeled vertebral renderings; **b** coronal and **c** sagittal spine renderings showing the complete plan after templating; **d** virtual plan model and **e** physical printed model of the templated spine

pedicle body. Based on this relationship, we define a the "Fastening Strength" as a surrogate for the screw holding power, which is estimated based on the virtually-templated images using the relationship below

$$Fastening\ Strength = \int_0^L \int_0^{2\pi} \int_0^{D/2} r \cdot I(r, \theta, z)\ dr\ d\theta\ dz, \qquad (1)$$

where L is the in-bone length of the screw, D is the screw diameter, and $I(r, \theta, z)$ is the image intensity of each voxel within bone volume displaced by the virtual screw. The above relationship represents the intensity—area product evaluated in transverse slices (defined by the in-plane cylindrical coordinates—radial distance r and angular increment $d\theta$) throughout the extent of the insertion depth L. This relationship is a surrogate primarily because the voxel intensity is used to characterize the bone mineral density (BMD) of the pedicle body segment displaced by the screw. Studies [11] have revealed a linear correlation between the image intensity and BMD measurements, based on calibrations of known BMD CaHA (calcium hydroxyapatite) phantoms against the dynamic intensity range: $BMD = \alpha \cdot Intensity$, where $\alpha = 0.8 \pm 0.03$. Moreover, the typical BMD of spinal cortical bone (hard shell coating the pedicle surface) was reported as $192 \pm 10\,\text{mg/cm}^3$ [12], which puts the cancellous bone (spongy bone near the pedicle core) BMD to $\sim 140\,\text{mg/cm}^3$.

The *Fastening Strength* however, *cannot* be interpreted as a widely-accepted absolute metric, but rather a relative measure to compare the approximate expected holding power provided by screws of different dimensions or implanted along different trajectories.

3 Initial Assessment of Spine Surgery Planning Platform

We conducted an initial assessment of the developed platform using retrospective clinical data from patients who underwent spine surgery that involve the implantation of pedicle screws. For the purpose of this study, we have limited our analysis to four cases, consisting of a total of 28 pedicle screws implanted in the lumbar spine of four patients. Procedures were performed using traditional planning (no use of the virtual planning platform) in the OR, based on standard pre-operative CT scans. Post-operative CT scans routinely ordered for follow-up purposes were used as ground truth (clinical gold standard) our assessment.

Several weeks after each procedure, a spine surgery fellow used the virtual platform to plan each procedure, resulting in a total of 36 virtual lumbar implants being suggested across all four cases. To enable paired assessment, only homologous implants (same vertebral level in both plan and procedure) were considered in the analysis, leading to a total of 26 paired implants.

3.1 Implant Dimension Assessment

The planned implant dimensions are automatically generated in the output report. To determine the dimensions of the screws implanted during the procedure, we used the virtual platform to "reverse plan" the post-operative CT along the lines of the screws present in the images (Fig. 3), and read the screw dimension from the output report. This approach allowed us to avoid any measurement uncertainties due to partial volume effects and beam hardening artifacts induced by the screws.

3.2 Implant Fastening Strength Assessment

The *Fastening Strength* of the planned implants was directly assessed by estimating the intensity—area product across the pedicel volume displaced by the virtually implanted screw. For post-operative assessment, each "reverse planned" vertebra was registered to its homologous counterpart in the pre-operative image (Fig. 4). Given the rigid individual vertebrae, an intensity-based rigid registration was used, followed

(a)   **(b)**

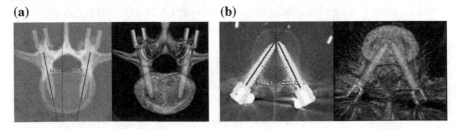

Fig. 3 Example of virtual templating and volume render representation at one vertebral segment. **a** Templating of pre-operative CT scan; **b** "reverse templating" of post-operative CT (high intensity metal implants are visible in the image)

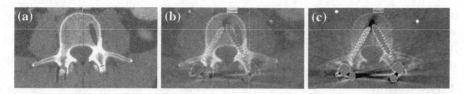

Fig. 4 Registration of post-operative "reverse plan" (**c**) to the pre-operaruve plan (**a**) for assessment of displaced bone volume to estimate *Fastening Strength*. The planned and actually inserted pedicle screws can be seen in the fused image (**b**)

Table 1 Summary of planned versus procedure measurements for implant diameter and length, as well as Fastening Strength, displaced bone volume, and mean voxel intensity of displaced bone volume

Measure	Screw diameter	Screw length	Fastening strength	Displaced bone volume	Mean Bone intensity
units	(mm)	(mm)	(mm$^3 \cdot$ HU)	(mm^3)	(HU)
Plan	5.5 ± 1.2	40.0 ± 2.0	$3.6 \cdot 10^7 \pm 0.7 \cdot 10^7$	$2.5 \cdot 10^3 \pm 0.4 \cdot 10^3$	164 ± 65
Procedure	6.9 ± 0.8	47.1 ± 5.0	$4.7 \cdot 10^7 \pm 0.8 \cdot 10^7$	$3.3 \cdot 10^3 \pm 0.5 \cdot 10^3$	167 ± 59

by minimal manual adjustment. Following registration, the intensity—area product was computed for each bone segment displaced by the post-operative implant.

Table 1 summarizes the implant dimension (diameter and length), the *Fastening Strength*, computed displaced bone volume, as well as its mean voxel intensity between the planned and actual procedure. While the average difference between the planned and implanted screws was on the order of 1 mm in diameter and 5 mm in length, the paired Student t-statistic revealed no difference between the parameters estimated from the virtual plan and actual procedure ($p > 0.01$), therefore suggesting that the results of planning platform are in agreement with the clinical gold standard.

Figure 5 compares the *Fastening Strength*, displaced bone volume, and mean voxel intensity of displaced bone volume between the plan and procedure. While no statistical difference was noted, the trend toward higher *Fastening Strength* achieved

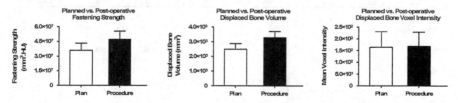

Fig. 5 Comparison between *Fastening Strength*, displaced bone volume and mean voxel intensity, showing no statistical difference ($p > 0.01$) between plan and procedure, therefore confirming consistency between the planned and clinical standard *Fastening Strength*

during the procedure correlated well with the trend toward larger displaced bone volume estimated from the pre-operative images, as well as with the slightly larger implants *versus*. plan.

4 Discussion

The relationship used to estimate the Fastening Strength is available in mechanical engineering compendia on machine component design and it was adapted to this application by relating the material strength to a surrogate measure of bone mineral density derived from CT image intensity. Given these estimates, we believe it is not critical to employ a complex finite element model under hypothetical loading conditions, especially given the current formulation suits any loading condition and provides a surrogate measure for the screw holding power. The fastening strength is computed based on the volume of bone displaced by the in-bone portion of the screw, assuming a cylindrical model whose diameter is measured across the thread, not just the screw shaft.

To further emphasize the consistency and utility of the *Fastening Strength* as a surrogate for the screw holding power, we performed further analyses on the observed *Fastening Strength*, displaced bone volume, and differences in implant dimension. Figure 6 illustrates the reduction in percent *Fastening Strength* with the decrease in screw dimension. As shown, as much as half of the holding power can be lost by undersizing the implant diameter by up to 3.5 mm, and as much as 35 % of the holding power can be lost by undersizing the implant length by up to 20 mm. These measurements are consistent with the displaced bone volume measurements relative to the implant dimension variability.

It is also worthwhile noticing that even for same dimension implants (no difference in diameter or length), uncertainties on the order of 3–5 % were observed in the displaced bone volume measurements, which, in turn, led to 5–10 % differences in holding power. While the difference in displaced bone volume measurements for identical size implants are artificial, primarily due to partial volume effects,

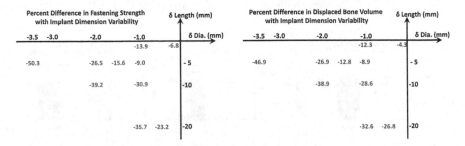

Fig. 6 percent difference in *Fastening Strength* and displaced bone volume with variations in implant dimension. The negative values indicate loss of holding power and underestimated displaced bone volume due to undersized implants

the remaining differences in *Fastening Strength* are real, and mainly due to the difference in voxel intensity within the displaced bone volume.

As far as mean voxel intensity within the displaced bone volume, the plan and procedure show comparable ranges, and moreover, consistent with the cancellous bone image intensity range. Recall that cortical spine BMD was estimated as $192 \pm 10 \, \text{mg/cm}^3$, while cancellous bone BMD at $\sim 140 \, \text{mg/cm}^3$; given the linear relationship between BMD and image intensity, cortical bone features a $\sim 235 \pm 14$ intensity range, while cancellous bone averages a mean voxel intensity of ~ 175. As shown in Table 1, the mean voxel intensity of the displaced bone volume in both the plan and procedure was on the order of 165 ± 60, which corresponds to the mean voxel intensity of cancellous bone, and moreover, extended into the lower limits of the cortical bone (~ 220). This, in fact, explains the wide variability of the measured mean voxel intensity in both the plan and procedure: while the screw shaft is immersed into the cancellous bone, the "tip of the thread" extends into the cortical bone surrounding the cancellous bone, toward the edge of the pedicle body.

According to our collaborating orthopedic surgeon, for a pedicle screw implant to be considered optimal, it is not only necessary for the screw to fully "tap" into the cancellous region, but the outer edges of the screw thread should "dig" into the hard cortical pedicle shell for improved holding power. Therefore, our proposed surrogate *Fastening Strength* metric fully supports this clinical requirement, and based on the mean voxel intensity measurements, the screws, in fact, fully "tapped" into the cancellous bone and also "grabbed" into the cortical bone, documented by the upper limits of the voxel intensity measurements.

While this approach may be interpreted as too simple, it provides consistent trends with screw size, within the limits defined by the clinical standard screw implantation procedures conducted with no computer assistance, chosen as gold standard for assessment of the plans. Claims that the proposed approach would be superior to the clinical standard would be very difficult to make, as they would invalidate the quality of health care provided via the clinical standard approach. Hence, we claim that the proposed approach provides objective measures for planning (i.e., screw dimensions, trajectory and holding power), and enables planning prior to the procedure and outside the OR, therefore leading to shorter procedures and time under anesthesia. We also demonstrated that the plans, within their inherent limitations introduced by the surgeon's skill level and screw measurement variability, provide similar fastening strength to the actual procedures. In addition, our surrogate *Fastening Strength* measure shows consistent trends with the screw size and correlates with the variations in the measured screw volume between the pre- and post-procedure data.

One limitation of the current study, besides the small sample size available for analysis, is the comparison of the virtual planning outcome to traditionally conducted procedures, therefore making it difficult to account for any potential deviations from the plan that could have occurred during the intervention. In addition, the retrospective virtual planning was performed by a (less experienced) fellow, while the actual procedures were performed by a senior surgeon, which explains the fellow's more conservative implant selection during planning—slightly thinner and shorter screws to avoid pedicle rupture or protrusion outside the vertebral body. To address these limitations, we intend to conduct a double cohort study that enables the translation of the plan into the OR for appropriate comparison of both virtual and traditional plans followed all the way to procedure outcomes. This study will also provide a larger sample size for analysis, and also enable us to study any differences between experienced and novice surgeons as far as implant selection and planning.

While other available computer-assisted spine intervention techniques are aimed at improving implant precision, such techniques make no effort to "remove the planning process" from the OR and minimize time under anaesthesia and overall procedure time. Since this platform allows planning to be performed once a pre-op CT scan is available, it is not counter-intuitive to conclude that by performing the planning prior to the procedure, the time under anesthesia, overall OR time and relates costs would be reduced.

5 Summary and Future Directions

We have described the development and initial clinical assessment of a spine surgery planning platform that integrates new and advanced visualization and planning via 3D virtual modeling and templating capabilities. As demonstrated by our analysis, while the platform leads to similar decisions as far as implant size selection, it allows surgeons to perform the planning *pre-operatively, outside of the OR* and rely on objective measures for safe and secure implant positioning. Results confirmed that *Fastening Strength* as a surrogate for holding power provides a rigorous metric for implant selection, as it accounts for both dimension and positioning, showing agreement between plan and procedure.

Future directions will involve further evaluation via both retro- and prospective studies, as well as the integration with existing computer-assisted orthopaedic surgery and navigation platforms [13], with the most obvious one being the Medtronic Stealth Station.

Acknowledgments The authors would like to thank all members of the Biomedical Imaging Resource who have helped with the development and implementation of this project, especially Alan Larson, Bruce Cameron, Phillip Edwards, and Dennis Hanson. Also, we would like to acknowledge our clinical collaborators for their continuous support: Dr. Jonathan Morris, Dr. Jane Matsumoto, and Dr. Shyam Shridharani.

References

1. Cohen M, Wall E, Brown R, Rydevik B, Garfin S (1990) Cauda equina anatomy II: extrathecal nerve roots and dorsal root ganglia. Spine 15:1248–1251
2. Rauschning W (1983) Computed tomography and cryomicrotomy of lumbar spine specimens: a new technique for multi-planar anatomic correlation. Spine (Phila Pa 1976) 8(2):170–180
3. Rauschning W (1987) Normal and pathologic anatomy of the lumbar root canals. Spine 12:1008–1019

4. Rydevik B, Brown M, Lundborg G (1984) Pathoanatomy and pathophysiology of nerve root compression. Spine 9:7–15
5. Wall E, Cohen M, Massie J, Rydevik B, Garfin S (1990) Cauda equine anatomy I: intrathecal nerve root organization. Spine 15:1244–1247
6. Hanson D, Robb RASA, Augustine KE, Cameron BM, Camp JJ, Karwoski RA, Larson AG, Stacy MC, Workman EL (1997) New software toolkits for comprehensive visualization and analysis of three-dimensional multimodal biomedical images. J Digit Imaging 10(Suppl. 1):229–230
7. Augustine K, Holmes III DR, Hanson D, Robb RA (2006) Comprehensive, powerful, efficient, intuitive: a new software framework for clinical imaging applications, pp 61,410N–10
8. Cameron BM, Manduca A, Robb RA (1996) Patient specific anatomic models: geometric surface generation from 3D medical images using a specified polygonal budget. In: Sieburg H, Weghorst S, Morgan K (eds) Health care in the information age. IOS Press and Ohmsha, pp 447–460
9. Lin WT, Robb RA (1999) Dynamic volume texture mapping and model deformation for visually realistic surgical simulation. Stud Health Technol Inform 62:198–204
10. Robb RA, Cameron BM, Aharon S (1997) Efficient shape-based algorithms for modeling patient specific anatomy from 3D medical images: applications in virtual endoscopy and surgery. In: Proceedings of the shape modeling and applications, pp 97–108
11. Homolka P, Gahleitner A, Prokop M, Nowotny R (2002) Bone mineral density measurement with dental quantitative CT prior to dental implant placement in cadaver mandibles: pilot study. Radiology 224(1):247–252
12. Jiang Y, Zhao J, Augat P, Ouyang X, Lu Y, Majumdar S, Genant HK (1998) Trabecular bone mineral and calculated structure of human bone specimens scanned by peripheral quantitative computed tomography: relation to biomechanical properties. Biomed Eng Online 13:1783–1790
13. Ortmaier T, Weiss H, Döbele S, Schreiber U (2006) Experiments on robot-assisted navigated drilling and milling of bones for pedicle screw placement. Int J Med Robot 2:350–363

Printed in the United States
By Bookmasters